They Call Me Harriet

They Call Me Harriet

My Life of Adventure, Romance,
and Molecular Biology

Harriet Latham Robinson

Copyright © 2024 by Harriet Latham Robinson

All rights reserved. No part of this publication may be reproduced, distributed, or transmitted in any form or by any means, including photocopying, recording, digital scanning, or other electronic or mechanical methods, without the prior written permission of the publisher, except in the case of brief quotations embodied in critical reviews and certain other noncommercial uses permitted by copyright law.

Published 2024
Printed in the United States of America
Print: 979-8-9910555-0-5
E-book: 979-8-9910555-1-2
Library of Congress Control Number: 2024915973

Cover and interior design by Tabitha Lahr
Cover photos © Courtesy of the author, and Shutterstock.com

To my beloved sons Bill, Al, and Tom

Disclosure

I have written my autobiography to the best of my memory coupled with the aid of my academic curriculum vitae, letters that my parents and in-laws saved, a diary kept between 2007 and 2014, my publications and my travel and presentation files. I sincerely apologize for any errors in this book. My cofounding of GeoVax resulted in my owning GeoVax stock, GeoVax warrants (expiring in 2025), and nonqualified GeoVax stock options (expiring in 2030). In January 2024, these represented less than 0.1 percent of the GeoVax market cap.

Contents

Disclosure... vii
Prologue.. xi

Part I: My Formative Years (1938–1962)

Chapter 1: My Boston Childhood (1938–1955) 3
Chapter 2: Learning Russian, Discovering Science, Summer Adventure (1955–1959)......... 15
Chapter 3: Guiding at the American Exhibition in Moscow (1959) 24
Chapter 4: Master's Degree in Biochemistry, Return to Russia (1959–1962)........... 38
Chapter 5: PhD Research on Messenger RNA (1962–1965).............................. 51
Chapter 6: Postdoctoral Training, and Marriage (1965–1967)............................. 57
Chapter 7: Early Marriage Years and Time Out for a Family (1967–1975) 64
Chapter 8: Return to Work (1975).................... 76
Chapter 9: Balancing the Lab and Family as a Single Parent (1977–1987) 89

Part II: My Academic Years (1977–2008)

Chapter 10: Cancer Induction by Insertional
              Mutagenesis (1977–1987) 109

Chapter 11: Pioneering Studies on DNA Vaccines
              (1989–1997) 120

Chapter 12: Research Toward an AIDS Vaccine
              Using Rabbit and Macaque Models
              (1989–2008) 134

Part III: My Entrepreneurial Years (2001–2019)

Chapter 13: Cofounding and Serving as Chief Scientific
              Officer of GeoVax (2001–2017) 151

Chapter 14: Development of GeoVax DNA and
              MVA HIV Vaccines (1998–2006) 160

Chapter 15: Clinical Trials of GeoVax's HIV
              Vaccines (2001–2019) 164

Epilogue: 2024 187
Acknowledgments 190
Glossary of Terms 192
Glossary of Key Contributors 202
About the Author 211

Prologue

I am writing my autobiography not only to recount my family story but to recount my scientific career where I was fortunate to have caught and ridden waves of findings in a new field— molecular biology. Molecular biology is the study of cellular molecules that carry out the biological processes that constitute life. All humans understand how the players in family life—mothers, fathers, sister, brothers, aunts, uncles—interact to give birth to and raise current and future generations. In contrast, most of us have only a superficial understanding, at best, of the molecules and the roles of the molecules that are basic players in molecular biology. In my story I explore the vital personal relationships that made me who I am as well as three of the players that are foundational to molecular biology. The first of these is deoxyribonucleic acid (DNA), the second is ribonucleic acid (RNA) and the third is protein. Below I tell the story not only of my life, but the story of my work as a molecular biologist with DNA, RNA, and protein.

I was blessed to have a life enriched by family as well as a profession. In part, I am writing my book to encourage women who are undertaking scientific careers to not forgo a family. Our best chance to naturally bear healthy children comes when we are in our twenties and early thirties. These are also the years that mark important rungs on the ladder for achieving tenure and leadership roles in science. The difference between bearing children and rising up professional ladders is that you can start up the ladder after you are forty. In contrast, motherhood is possible, but much more problematic, after forty.

And finally, my title, *They Call Me Harriet*. At scientific symposia and committee meetings, the male participants would be referred to as "doctor" so and so or "professor" so and so. In contrast, I was Harriet. I was content to be an active, albeit first-name participant; but it would have been nice to have had more formal recognition.

PART I:
My Formative Years (1938–1962)

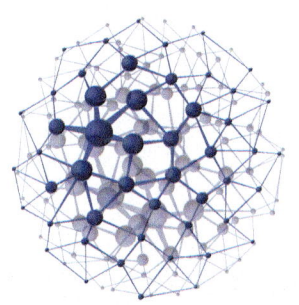

CHAPTER 1:

My Boston Childhood (1938–1955)

Snow was falling on the night of my birth, February 10, 1938. My father drove our black Buick across the less drifted side yard to get my mother to the hospital on time. I was the second of four children; Nick was two years older and David and Tom would be born two and five years later. My paternal grandparents were particularly pleased at my arrival. I was their tenth grandchild and the first girl. My grandfather had made a special chair for a female grandchild. It had tooled rungs and a woven rush seat. Bearing the chair, Grandad and Grandma Latham drove from Connecticut to Boston to admire me. My "big" brother, Nick, called me HeyHey and pronounced that I smelled.

I had been spawned by educated and happy parents. My mother, Ruth Nichols, was an Ohio girl from Medina, a town south of Cleveland, with the road sign declaring it HOG CAPITAL OF THE WORLD. Her father, a dentist, took care of his hog farmers, accepting produce as pay, if necessary. She loved her horse, Topsy, and was valedictorian of her high school class. She was interested in science, majoring in chemistry at Oberlin, where she received both a bachelor's and a master's degree. Following Oberlin, she accepted a position as an instructor in chemistry at Smith College. She found the Smith Chemistry Department populated by unhappy women obsessed with the details of how to lay out their equipment rather than the chemical reactions they were studying. After Smith, my mother's view was that "an educated woman could not be a happy woman."

My father, Allen Latham Jr., was from Norwichtown Connecticut. He was the son of a beekeeper and high school science teacher. His father's sister, Aunt Azubah, had risen through the academic ranks of Columbia University to chair the Department of Speech. Aunt Azubah had an apartment on the Upper West Side of New York City that my father loved to visit. She created sufficient wealth that she helped pay my father's college tuition and in her will requested that if he had a daughter, that she be named Harriet (after her mother) and be college educated. I am that daughter.

My parents met at a dance in Charleston, West Virginia where my father and my mother's brother, Ab—both young engineers—were employed by DuPont. Following her Smith experience, my mother had returned to Medina where she was making beeswax candles at the Root Co. Ab had invited his sister, ready to move on from her time at Smith, for a West Virginia weekend and dance. My father was smitten by the visiting sister, whom he remembers as wearing a flowing yellow dress. My mother remembers my father as attractive, but smoking (a no-no). The next morning my father lost no time in visiting Ab, where he found my mother on the front porch, brushing her hair and swinging with Ab's toddlers. She passed him a toddler. My father never smoked again. Their marriage at the Medina family home came a few months later, on Armistice Day, and is memorialized in a film. As a wedding gift, my father gave his bride an ivory hairbrush, comb, and mirror. The wedding film is still with us, and particularly entertaining when shown backward.

The newlyweds settled in Charleston where my father continued his job at DuPont. Tragedy struck when Ab, working on a Sunday, was killed by a chemical explosion. He had come out from behind the safety shield to adjust equipment. In the effort to save his life, my father directly donated blood by gravity flow. The incident left a lasting impression on my father, both in how poorly DuPont supported the widow and in the need for better blood processing. DuPont took no responsibility for Ab's family other than his final paycheck. The widow, with an infant and two toddlers, all girls, returned to Medina where my maternal grandparents helped raise Ab's children. My father, in his later years, would develop blood processing equipment, equipment that might have saved Ab, had it been available.

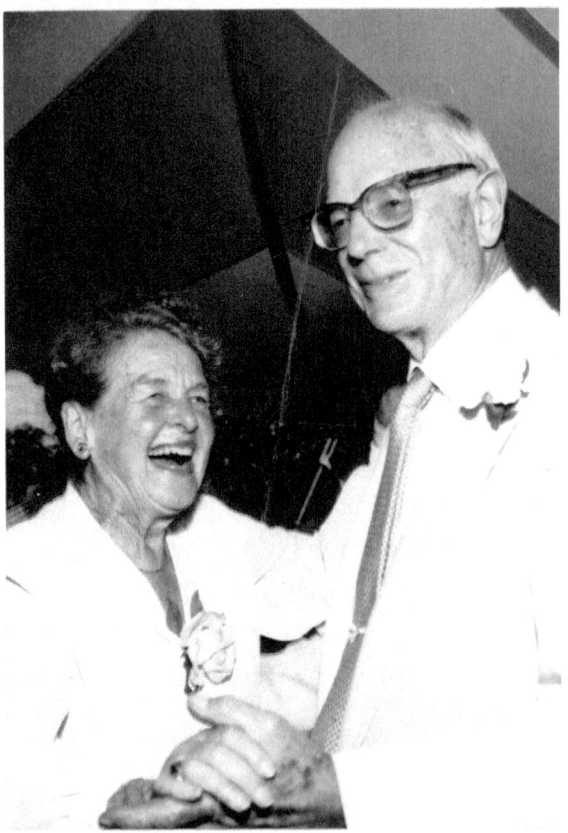

My Parents. My parents enjoying each other's company as they dance at their eldest grandson's wedding. Over their marriage, my parents successfully developed interests together. In exchange for my father attending the opera, which he grew to like, my mother learned how to cope with her seasickness to sail with my father.

My parents left West Virginia in 1935 for Boston when DuPont entered my father into the newly formed MIT Sloan Fellows Program, a business program for engineers with potential for general management. While my father's career advanced, my mother devoted herself to being a housewife and having children.

Our home in Jamaica Plain, a Boston neighborhood, backed onto acres of fields, hills, woods, and ponds left over from the weekend estates of clipper ship captains who lived on Beacon Hill. After school, I spent hours with Poochy, the family dog, roaming the estates. In the winter, we followed the tracks in the snow of squirrels, rabbits, dogs, and pheasants while we sledded, tobogganed, and skated. In the spring, we watched the pollywogs become frogs, flushed pheasants, and discovered where birds were nesting. After chicks had fledged, I collected the nests, which in junior high would win me second place in the City of Boston Science Fair. This win, coming from Poochy's and my adventures, would be the first recognition of my interest in science, an interest that blossomed over my lifespan.

When I reached school age, the age for starting kindergarten had been reduced from five to four to free mothers to fill needed jobs in support of World War ll. My older brother, Nick, proudly took me, with my new umbrella, to visit the Joseph P. Manning school. This public school had a single grade per room for first and sixth grade but two grades per room for second through fifth grades. The Boston Public Library supplied books and magazines at the back of the rooms, which one could read when assignments were completed and the other grade was being taught. I particularly enjoyed Dr. Dolittle books and the *National Geographic* magazines. Recess, which I loved, allowed us to go outside to a surfaced play area where the boys and girls had separate kickball games and the girls jumped rope.

My only regular after school activities were piano lessons, which I tolerated, and delivering the *Jamaica Plain Citizen*, a weekly newspaper, which Poochy, my friend Martha and her dog Misty, and assorted other neighborhood dogs (who could not resist joining us) delivered on Thursdays. It was easier delivering the newspapers than collecting the monthly dues. I rang certain doorbells with trepidation about the social interaction that was about to take place. Fortunately, most of the households readily paid their bills.

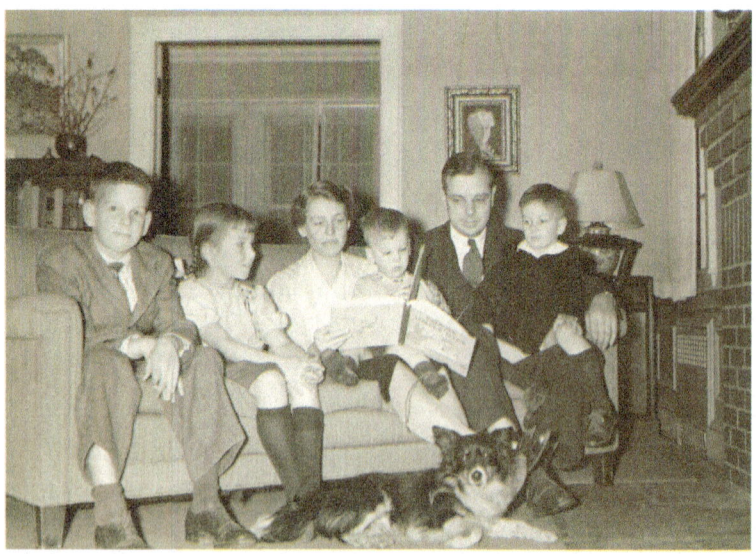

1946 Christmas Picture of the Latham Family. From left to right, Nick, me, my mother holding Tom, and my father holding Dave. Poochy is lying on the floor in front of her family.

World War II spanned my early life, beginning in 1939 when I was a toddler and ending in 1945 when I was in second grade. Outside of rationing, blackouts, and my being afraid that Hitler would nab me in our basement when I was sent to get a jar of canned tomatoes, life during World War II was remarkably tranquil. Sugar, gas, and tires were rationed. The lack of sugar meant we could not make jelly or can as many peaches as my mother would have liked. The lack of tires and gas meant that driving was limited to absolutely essential trips. We collected fat left over from cooking and donated it for use in the manufacture of explosives. My father's engineering skills were redirected to the manufacture of war machinery. There was a pile of metal cylinders for compressed gasses, called skinks, that looked like oversized bombs in our backyard. We were strictly forbidden to play with the skinks. When we went to the beach, we carefully avoided flotsam and jetsam that could contain unexploded ordnance. Outside of the brother of one of our favorite babysitters being killed by friendly fire while on night patrol in Germany, we experienced little of the death and maiming of the war.

Travel was limited because of the gas rationing and the inability to get tires. Our "non-car" adventure was to take the Steel Pier, a ferry that ran from Boston to Provincetown. Provincetown is where the Pilgrims first landed. At Provincetown we would bicycle to Race Point, the very tip of Cape Cod, and camp in the sand dunes. The first year just my father, Nick, and I went, Nick on the second seat of a rented tandem bike and me on a seat that my father had built over the luggage carrier. By the next year, I had the second seat of the tandem, David was on the luggage carrier, and Nick had his own bike. In the final year, my mother and Tom joined us. We carried everything we needed in backpacks and biked into town every night for hot fudge sundaes. We would use coals from our cooking fire to warm the sand around our blankets before going to bed. We were camping in the dunes when bells, sirens, and fireworks announced Victory Japan Day and the end of World War II. At age seven, I was jubilant and celebrated with my father, Nick, and David in the sand dunes of Race Point.

Once the war was over, my family acquired an army surplus jeep and army surplus sleeping bags and tents. My father mounted the spare tire for the jeep across the back opening to prevent our falling out and built a wooden seat between the two front seats. All six of us and our gear could fit. When hitchhikers would hold out a thumb for a ride, my brothers and I would yell "no vacancies." We took the jeep to Race Point, but the main camping destinations were New Hampshire, Vermont, and Canada. We did a remarkable amount of hiking, even making the top of Mount Washington, the 6,289-foot tallest peak in New England. They were simple, but happy family times.

In 1949, when I graduated from grammar school and was ready for junior high and high school, I, then twelve years old, entered Girls' Latin School, a public magnet school for the college-bound young women of Boston. It was a rigorous school excelling in language and history that took its students through twelfth grade. There was no science, outside of Miss Lord's health class and one year of chemistry. It had no school library, limited athletic facilities, and essentially no support of the arts except for glee and drama clubs. Despite its limitations, Girls' Latin School, which my father called "Miss Lord's finishing off school for young girls," provided a remarkable education. Its lack of physical facilities was more than made up for by its teachers, who prided themselves on teaching at Latin School. When I got to college, I could take Russian because of my score in the College Board Latin exam. Miss O'Conner and the passion with which she taught ancient and European history founded my lifelong love of history.

The Latin School student body represented the diversity of Boston and its neighborhoods. A disproportionate number of the students (about 30 percent) were from Boston's Jewish community. I soon had Jewish as well as Christian friends. We visited each other's homes and places of worship. My first wine was at my friend Roz's synagogue at the Saturday morning service. It was part of the ceremony. I was jolted by the unexpected taste, so different from the grape juice used in ceremonies at my church. In later years, when Roz was married, I was awed by the celebratory atmosphere, which not only included smashing the wine glass but a wolf whistle for the bride's mother (who was gorgeous in a shining sheath) as she came down the aisle. Roz's wedding was a total contrast to the chaste seven-minute protestant service of my church.

At our fiftieth and sixtieth high school reunions, I was struck by what my Girls' Latin School classmates had done with their lives. We had become not only the wives, mothers, teachers, and nurses we were supposed to become, but also, physicians, lawyers, professors, politicians, and businesswomen. Many of us played leadership roles in our communities. Girls' Latin had provided an academic foundation that we could build on. But, equally important, by being an all-girls school, it had provided a social setting in which we were not dominated by adolescent males. In my very male family, outside of my mother being the social secretary, men led. Attending an all-girls school during my adolescence, a place where boys did not lead, encouraged and allowed me to think independently.

During my junior high years, my mother became bedbound with headaches. There was no diagnosis until my father, having exhausted the experts of the Boston medical community, turned back to Dr. Marlow, the family doctor. Dr. Marlow administered a careful physical, including a reflex exam, and realized that her right knee was overresponding to the hammer tap. Overresponse of a knee reflex can be an indicator of a brain tumor. It turned out that my mother had a meningioma. Meningiomas grow on the surface of the brain and are operable. My father brought Sadie, a second cousin, from the Maine woods, to help with the family. The first surgery successfully removed the tumor and a second installed a metal plate where her skull had been removed. A neighbor, who was a nurse, stayed with my mother for the immediate postoperative period. We children were not allowed to visit her in the hospital, although she could wave to us from a window, where we were reassured and excited to see her.

I don't remember how my father told us of the tumor and impending surgery. I do remember that my father (an engineer) approached her illness as something that could be fixed. He let us know that our mother had a tumor, but conveyed confidence that it was an operable tumor. I went to school on the day of the surgery and the school told me of the successful completion of the surgery.

I remember my father preparing us for my mother's homecoming from the hospital. For the first few months, my mother would need an adult with her at all times should she have a seizure while her brain expanded to occupy the space left by the tumor. My father held a family meeting at which he served peanuts. At the meeting, we discussed my mother's homecoming and my father let us know about the risk of seizures.

We then discussed what we, the children, should do if she seized. Rather than leaving us to be terrified in the event of a seizure, my father told us that seizures are a normal part of recovery from surgical removal of a meningioma and explained exactly what to do should she have a seizure. We were to help the adult get her lying down and to put a spoon in her mouth to prevent her biting her tongue. Thankfully, my mother had a seizure-free recovery. But, although completely functional, my mother never completely recovered her original self. She could keep house and lead an active social life. She maintained her enthusiasm and still liked to go places and do things. In later years, she traveled with me in Europe and helped with the babies when I had children. When my spouse developed life-threatening septicemia, initiated by a rose thorn, right before Christmas, I called my in-laws. They were leaving for the holidays to visit family and responded that they would call once they were in Mississippi. I then called my parents. My mother was on the next plane to California to come and help me (I had three small children).

As my high school years progressed, my father played an ever more central role in my life. Despite my mother's absolute dedication to her husband and children, her post-surgery antennae did not pick up teenage woes. When I dragged my heels about going to Miss Souther's ballroom dancing class, she sent me to my room with no supper. My father, concerned about what was going on at dancing school, rescued me from my closet. He rapidly realized that no one was dancing with me. His solution was to send me and my mother to get me a new dress. My mother had bought my "dancing school" dress from a friend. It was a poorly fitting mustard-yellow dress that the friend had made from expensive wool and that neither the friend's daughter nor I wanted to wear. After her surgeries, my mother did not have the social intuition to ask why I did not want to go to dancing school, but she did have the ability to enthusiastically execute my father's solution of a new dress. Together we picked a beautiful red velvet dress. The new dress worked.

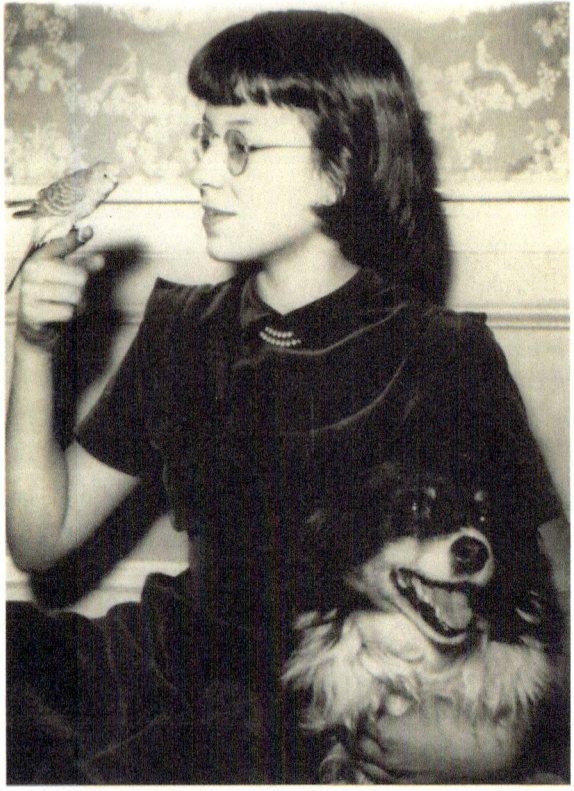

The Red Velvet Dress. A black and white picture of me in my wonderful red velvet dress. My parakeet Jasper is on my finger and Poochy is at my side. Jasper had a more than twenty-word vocabulary and could wolf whistle.

CHAPTER 2:

Learning Russian, Discovering Science, Summer Adventure (1955–1959)

As I grew older, I received advice from both parents. I most clearly remember the advice from my mother as I boarded the train for college. "Don't study," she said. She, burned by her year at Smith, was warning me against overeducation setting the stage for being an unhappy spinster, or at best an unhappy homemaker. My goal for college should be to find the right husband, not train for a profession. I remembered my mother's advice but did not take it. I was not a bookworm, but I did study at college. College courses opened new vistas for me. In mathematics, there was calculus and the handling of multiple numbers over an interval to determine a whole. In economics, I learned that deficit spending could prime an economic pump. Deficit spending was totally foreign to my New England sensibility that one never spent more than what one had. For me, exposure to the world and the knowledge that man has accumulated over the centuries is one of the great treats of life.

It had been the tradition in my mother's family to attend Oberlin. The Ohio family valued Oberlin, because from its very beginning in 1833, it had educated African Americans and women, as well as men. I also applied to Swarthmore, a small Quaker college. Accepted at both, I chose Swarthmore. I had liked a student play that was performed the weekend that I visited. I also liked that Swarthmore, on a commuter train line to Philadelphia, was much less isolated than Oberlin.

Essentially simultaneous with my arrival by train from Boston, my freshman roommate, Jan, arrived by train from Omaha. Looking back, we realized we had both been on the same local commuter train connecting us from the Philadelphia station to Swarthmore. We looked at each other, took off our hats and gloves and went to college. Both of us were able students. Jan was a science major with an interest in biology. I was a political science major with an interest in languages. Freshman year, I took biology to fulfill my requirement for a course in science. An enthusiastic young professor taught Introductory Biology. He presented both plant and animal kingdoms and then showed us how in the animal kingdom the development of embryos recapitulated the simple to more complex forms of life in the evolutionary tree. For example, human embryos in their very early stages of development have gills not unlike those in current fish. I was fascinated by how single cells replicated and built on patterns of development as they became diverse multicellular organisms, a phenomenon that is now known to reflect cross-species conservation of genes for development.

By the end of the year, I had switched my major from political science, where the Introductory Course had seemed like a lot of platitudes, to a new and exciting field for me, biology.

Whereas political science became supplanted by biology, my interest in languages held. At Girls' Latin, we had skipped the chapter in our *American Studies* book with the portrait of a smiling Stalin. The book had been written at the close of World War II when the United States and Russia were allies. Because it was left out of our assignments, the chapter about Russia piqued my curiosity. Why should Stalin have gone from being presented as a smiling ally to being purposefully omitted? By speaking and reading Russian I would be less at the mercy of reporters and textbook authors who were switching their opinions from one year to the next. It would also be in keeping with my interest in political science, my major when I started Introductory Russian.

Russian at Swarthmore was taught by Miss Lamkirt, an émigré who had been a lady in waiting to the last tsarina, a granddaughter of Queen Victoria. At the start of the 1917 revolution Miss Lamkirt had escaped through China, where she supported herself doing secretarial work before coming to the United States in 1949 when the Communists, led by Mao Tse-tung, took over mainland China. There were three students in our pre-Sputnik Russian class: me, a student named Peter, and an astronomy professor, also named Peter. As we learned Russian grammar, Miss Lamkirt taught us folk songs and children's rhymes which we sang and recited. We used our new vocabulary and grammar, no matter how limited, to write her a story a week. At the end of the lesson, she served Russian honey cake. This remarkable training, by an erstwhile member of the Russian nobility, would land me a job as a Russian-English speaking guide at the 1959 American National Exhibition in Moscow.

A lasting gift Swarthmore gave me was Jan. Not only did we room together freshman year, but we remained roommates for the next three years. At the end of our college years, Jan received a prestigious Marshall Scholarship to study genetics at the University of Edinburgh. From the moment she got off the plane in Scotland, she was "at home" and has remained in Scotland ever since. When I hit a personal crisis in my graduate school years, and was in an unhappy engagement, I went to visit Jan over Christmas vacation and came back healed, able to go forward. Her daughter is named after me. In our later years we traveled together—to India, China, Israel, southern Spain and Machu Picchu. She has been and still is a true and deep friend.

When I was finishing college, the appropriate next steps for a properly educated young lady were marriage, becoming a nurse, or becoming a teacher. Not having a marriage prospect, I opted to become a teacher and applied to the master's program at the Harvard Graduate School of Education. At my interview, I sought permission to replace courses in education with courses in science. The woman interviewing me shunted me and my request up the admissions office bureaucracy. I eventually landed in the office of a Radcliffe dean, who, after listening to my request to take science instead of education courses said, "My dear, you want to be a scientist, not a teacher." This woman, to whom I am forever grateful, not only recognized my interest in science but considered it perfectly appropriate for a young woman to become a scientist. On the spot, she provided me with the forms to apply to the Harvard Graduate Program in Biochemistry. I also applied to MIT—in both cases seeking a master's degree.

Learning Russian, Discovering Science, Summer Adventure

Harvard, a mature program, was biased toward students seeking doctoral degrees and turned me down. MIT was just beginning the expansion of its program in biological sciences, a program that is now among the most productive in the world and was open to master's candidates. I was accepted by MIT and offered a fellowship to teach the Introductory Biology lab to pay my way. I immediately accepted the fellowship and was excited to have the opportunity to be preparing for a career in science, not education.

Instead of doing summer internships, my summers were times of outdoor adventure. Following my freshman year at Swarthmore, I was a biking counselor at a sailing camp on Martha's Vineyard. Following my sophomore and junior years, I was a hiking counselor in California at Camp Timberloft, just outside the south gate of Yosemite National Park. During her Oberlin years, my mother, as part of an ecology course, had camped across the western United States. By some miracle, she and my father agreed that I, with two Swarthmore friends, and under the condition that we had summer jobs, could take a car west. The three of us promptly found summer jobs in California. In preparation for the trip, my father had me practice changing a tire and setting up the tent. He also counseled me that when pulling onto a turnpike, one had to be sure to allow sufficient room in front of the oncoming cars to get up to turnpike speed. I was not to use the car to tow anything and I was to call in nightly with our location.

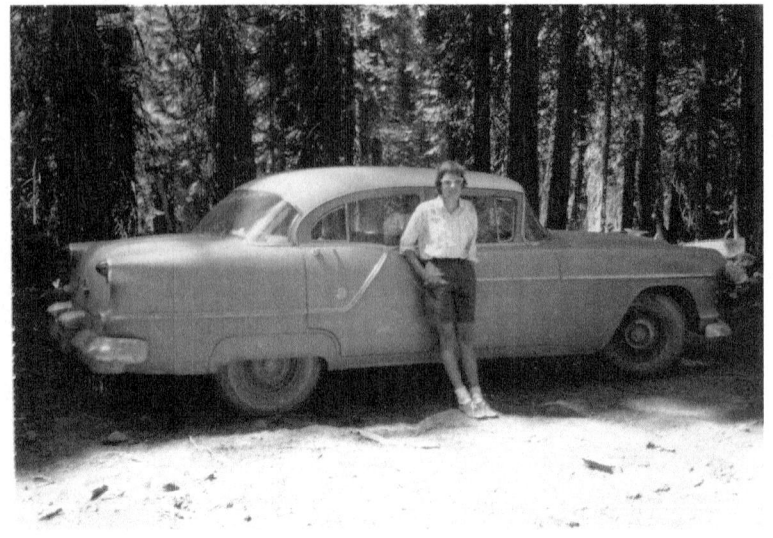

The Turquoise Body, white-top Oldsmobile. Nineteen years old, I am standing by the car in Yosemite.

We set out in early June, two weeks before our jobs were to start. I was at the wheel carefully steering, so as not to hit the Mass Turnpike toll booth. Once past the booth, I purposefully powered the car up to turnpike speed. Our first night on the road was at Swarthmore where students were finishing up exams. We slept in the dorm and ate in the cafeteria. The next night we were in Ohio, where we stayed at the third camper's home. Now we were truly on our way. The fourth night we camped in a public campground. The heavens let loose. We hastily dragged picnic tables under a gazebo and slept on the tables. Traveling before Eisenhower's interstate highways, we were making 250 to 300 miles a day, rotating the driver at two-hour intervals. When we got to New Mexico, we stayed with my Aunt Barbie and Uncle Howard, professional artists. We slept among the easels in Barbie's studio. Before heading west again,

Barbie served us an enormous poached egg breakfast. By the day before I was to start my job, we reached Death Valley. There, we camped in the Furnace Creek Campground. It was hot. We sprinkled water on our sleeping bags to cool by evaporation, and promptly became too cold. The solution was to get up and drive on, pulling into California at dawn. Looking at the map, we decided to head north on the east side of the Sierras and cross the Sierras using the Tioga Pass road.

Unbeknownst to us, Tioga Pass closes for the winter, but fortunately for us, had just reopened. As we turned onto the pass, there was a sign: Tioga Pass—Open. Soon, enormous piles of snow lined the single-lane road. Pull-offs allowed snow-moving equipment to let the only car on the road pass: an Oldsmobile from Massachusetts, with three teenage girls inside. Dazzled by the snow, we threaded our way into Tuolumne Meadows, unpacked our jackets and fixed some breakfast. From there it was only six hours to Timberloft, where Porky, the camp director, was a bit taken aback that we had come in over Tioga Pass.

Early the next morning, I deposited my co-adventurers at the Fresno bus station to continue to their summer jobs in San Francisco and Santa Cruz and returned to camp in time for the start of counselor training. On our cross-country trip, we had had no major snafus, no flat tires. We had been surprised by the amount of snow in the western mountains and the heat of Death Valley. Downpours had drenched us but had not washed us away. We had made it.

Timberloft had a lodge/kitchen and a swimming pool but no cabins or dining hall. Units slept together in clustered "nests" framed with logs and filled with pine needles. My unit, the Rangers, nested way out in the woods. At first, I had trouble finding the Rangers' nests at night and would return to the sound of the camp generator to make a second attempt. Girls would come for two-week sessions. The first few days they would acclimatize (we were at about five thousand feet) while we did day hikes.

By far the most adventurous day hike we did was the famed Yosemite Valley Half Dome. This sixteen-mile round trip hike with a 4800-foot gain in elevation has cables (then chains) anchored in granite for the last ascent. Part of our group opted to stay with the assistant counselor at a spring right before the final ascent. The rest of us made the top. One of the fathers had written that his daughter should be careful not to be stressed. This girl vomited at the top of Half Dome. I felt tremendously responsible that I had not remembered the father's concern and let his daughter go for the top. But the daughter, ecstatic, was totally upbeat about the ascent, both before and after her stomach objected. By not remembering the father's warning, I may have let her undertake an adventure that her family would not have let her have! It was late when we started down. Some backpackers fed us chicken soup as we passed little Yosemite Valley. When we reached the valley floor, I bought pints of ice cream for everyone and called camp that we would be late getting home. Porky, worried, was hovering in the camp drive as the cattle truck pulled in just after 10:00 p.m. I was never afraid, nor were the girls. They were tired but triumphant at what they had done. It was an amazing hike!!!

Sessions would end with a four-to-five-day backpacking trip in the Yosemite or King's Canyon high country. There, we made the classical, as well as less classical, loops, camping under the stars, scaring off the bears by shaking pebbles in

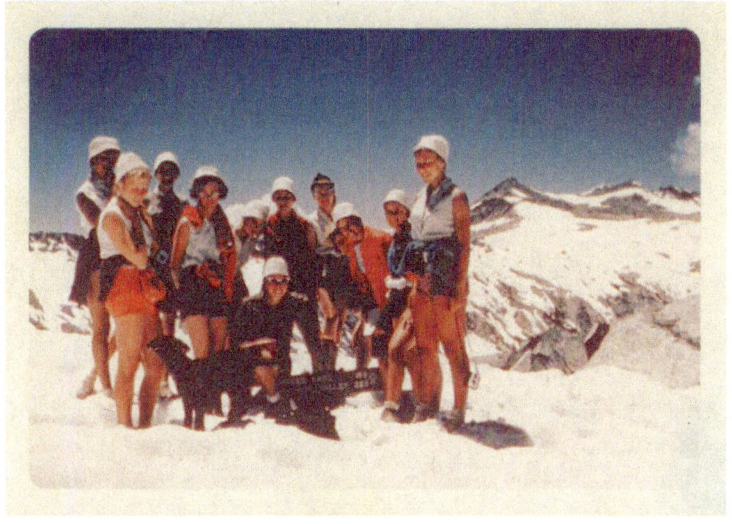

Granite Pass. Here is where we turned back from going to Red Peak Pass because of the snow. I am sitting on the trail sign that is showing just above the snow. The dog belonged to my assistant counselor who took the picture.

tin cans, heating rocks to warm our sleeping bags. We drank from the streams and made snow cones from the glaciers. I became an expert at treating blisters and by my second year was sending pre-camp letters to families on the importance of sturdy shoes. The one hike we never succeeded in making was over Red Peak Pass, where snow turned us back. They were wonderful summers.

CHAPTER 3:

Guiding at the American Exhibition in Moscow (1959)

In the spring of 1959, my senior year at Swarthmore, plans for exchange exhibitions between the Soviets and the Americans were featured on the front page of the *New York Times*. The Soviet exhibit was to be in New York City, and the American exhibit, in Moscow. I was interested in history and politics. It was a time of political thaw between Russia and the United States. I had spent four years learning Russian. It was a golden opportunity. I wrote to the name in the article, inquiring whether there might be a job for a Russian-English speaking guide and received an invitation to interview in DC. My then Russian teacher (Miss Lamkirt had retired), helped me prepare answers, in Russian, to likely questions. On March 17, I put on my beige knit suit, took the train to DC, and interviewed. They did ask the expected questions and I did my best with unexpected questions like "how much does a cab driver make?"—which I answered with how much the minister of my church made, the only salary I knew outside of what counselors at Girl Scout camps made.

I got the job, with my name being written by hand at the end of an alphabetized list of the typed names of the other guides. My handwritten name out of alphabetical order, meant I had been a last-minute addition. It had been a squeaker. But unlike most of the guides, I was not the child of an émigré or trained by the military at the Monterey language school. Rather, I had been born in Massachusetts and had parents from Ohio and Connecticut. I had gone to public schools and worked at Girl Scout camps. I represented a very ordinary American. Where I was atypical was that I had taken four years of Russian in college.

The seventy-five guides, between eighteen and thirty-five years old, consisted of twenty-eight females and forty-seven males. We first assembled on June 15 at the Presidential Hotel in DC where we were unexpectedly loaded onto military buses and transported to the White House. Cleared through security, we were led to the Oval Office to meet President Eisenhower. The Oval Office was smaller than I expected and Ike was shorter than I expected. Ike, skillfully cordial, came out from behind his desk to greet us. He spoke briefly on the importance of the exhibition to Soviet-American relations and to the importance of our representing America to the best of our abilities at this historic exchange of exhibits. He congratulated the two African American members of our staff. The meeting was followed by a photo in the Rose Garden. We reboarded the buses to be flown by military aircraft to New York City for three days at the Fashion Institute where the sewing machines hummed, fitting the women in five red, white, and blue "on duty" outfits. These outfits had been chosen by fashion experts to display the type of clothes worn by everyday Americans. The male outfits were red sports shirts paired with navy blue jackets, and gray flannel slacks. The women could choose which outfit they wore each day. The style, the color and our large guide buttons readily identified us to Soviet visitors.

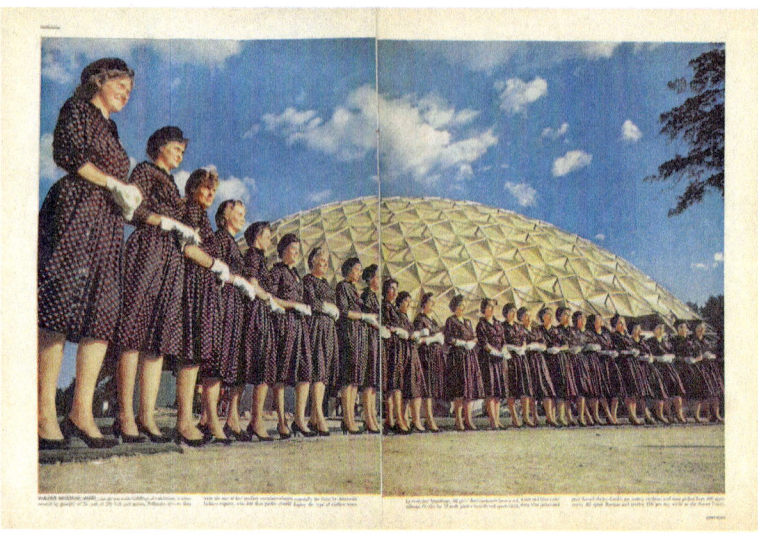

Female Guides at the American Exhibition in Moscow. This picture was taken by Life Magazine on the day of the opening. We are in our "dress" uniforms and arranged by height. I am seventh in from the right. The Geodesic Dome, one of the two main buildings at the Fair is in the background.

Training for the upcoming exhibition started with a general introduction on the evening of the fifteenth. This was followed on the sixteenth and seventeenth by panel discussions and question-and-answer periods addressing "Soviet Approaches to Information" and "Meeting Russians." On June 18, we boarded a chartered train to Montreal, where we would sail for Genoa on June 19. During twelve days aboard the *Irpinia*, training continued with language drills, a review of American civilization and practice sessions answering questions. On July 2, we debarked in Cannes (there was a strike in Genoa) to travel by train for overnights in Milan, Nuremberg, Prague, and Warsaw before arriving in Moscow on July 7.

We crossed the Iron Curtain marked by barbed wire, watchtowers, and plowed fields between West Germany and Czechoslovakia, where we stopped to get our passports cleared in a train yard filled with slogans: FORWARD TO SOCIALISM, LIFE WITH COMMUNISM. I saw women, bent over, wearing dark kerchiefs—a sinister image—sweeping the tracks with short-handled brooms, and trains, with large red stars on the steam engines, pulling in and out. And then, suddenly, a train full of Russian youth pulled alongside us and, leaning out of the windows, we started talking to each other.

"Where are you from?"

"America," I said.

"Moscow," they said.

"I am working at the US Exhibition," I said.

"We are going to a youth festival," they said.

"We are so glad you came," they said and as their train began to pull out, they threw cigarettes and candies to us and those of us who had something to throw threw gifts to them. And then, somehow, I knew we were there, and that behind the Iron Curtain were going to be people with whom I could talk, people with whom I could be moved to spontaneous giving.

In Prague and Warsaw, we stayed in dormitories where local students toured us and gave us the first taste of the questions we would face as guides. In Prague we first saw spontaneous queues to buy goods. Later in Moscow, we would see Soviets queue while they figured out what was being sold. Would it be apples, books, toilet paper? In stores, vegetables and canned goods were a rarity and shoes exorbitant, yet there were signs advertising new TV sets. There were new stadiums, reflecting the emphasis on sports of the Communist regime.

In contrast to Italy and West Germany, where rebuilding from World War II had been largely completed, there was active rebuilding, especially in Poland. The Poles hated the Germans and still feared loss of their land. When we crossed the Polish border, the gauge of our train was changed and the German maps at the ends of cars substituted with Polish maps showing the Polish, not the German version, of Polish-German borders.

After a day in Warsaw, and a visit to the Warsaw ghetto, we were on to Moscow on the overnight train, four of us to a compartment, the porter bringing us tea in glasses. When the train stopped in Minsk for an hour, I walked to the center of town with Herb, our six-foot-four African American guide who was wearing his blue sunglasses. The residents of Minsk gawked, practically fell over. They had never seen a real live African American, never mind a truly tall one parading in blue sunglasses. Once in Russia we saw constant billboards: Peace and Friendship, Communism means Electrification. As we pulled into Moscow, baggage was sorted for the last time. We were each traveling with 100 pounds including spring through fall clothing and our American fashion outfits. Buses took us to the Ostankino Hotel on the outskirts of Moscow, which had been chosen for its proximity to Solkoniki Park where the exhibition was located. We settled into our rooms with our assigned roommates. The rooms, standard hotel rooms, were under the watchful eyes of women who sat at tables on each floor and controlled the keys. The curtains were lace. The blankets, down puffs.

It was only ten days until opening and the preparation of the exhibit was three weeks behind schedule. Further orientation was cancelled so that we could help the US contractors and embassy staff get the exhibit open on time. The one exception to work unpacking, assembling, and cleaning was Russian lessons, which continued for those of us with weaker language skills, which included me!

The Soviets were busy with landscaping. To my astonishment, women were moving dirt in hand-carried wooden litters and cutting lawns (large lawns) with hand shears. When asked by Soviets what had surprised me most in Moscow, this was my answer at first. Seeing the disappointment in their eyes and the stoop in their shoulders, though, I learned not to give this answer. Russians were proud of how they were rebuilding their country from World War II and doing the best they could with what they had. If one wanted to go onto further meaningful conversation, the answer, a very honest answer, was that I was most surprised by the pride the Russian people took in the post-World War II accomplishments of their country.

As soon as we were through work for the day, we would take the streetcar to downtown Moscow where we found every restaurant with the exact same menu, limited napkins, and water glasses that were not changed between diners. The standard menu was the same as had been in the dining car on the train into Moscow. It had soups such as borscht and solyanka, blini (thin pancakes), piroshki (meat hand pies), caviar, steak with a fried egg on top, and chicken Kiev (deep fried chicken stuffed with melting garlic butter—my favorite). Vegetables, except for green peas, were nonexistent. The bread, Russian potato bread, was delicious. Not all items on this standard menu were available. Except for a few specialty restaurants, food was very mediocre in its preparation. Restaurants and stores used abacuses for checkout. At grocery or department stores, one stood in line to get the price of an item, then stood in line to pay and get a payment chit, and then, with the payment chit, stood in line to pick up one's purchase. One carried one's purchases in string bags which folded up to nothing when not in use. There were no cash registers and payments for goods were going into drawers with little accounting activity. If I had been given one reform I could have brought to the Soviets, it would have been cash registers.

At the fairground, exhibits were taking shape and the Soviet band was practicing "The Star-Spangled Banner." And then, we were open, Khrushchev and Nixon gave speeches, and the elite of Moscow, dressed in their good clothes, paraded through the exhibits. I manned my exhibit, a US playground, which I likely had been assigned because it required less skill in the Russian language than more controversial exhibits such as the ranch-style "typical" American home and modern art.

On the next day, the first working day of the exhibit, the public flooded in. Not all signs were up, the cement went to pieces on the floors of the two main buildings, and the books were being lifted so fast that US and Moscow security guards, working together, could not stem the outflow. We guides worked six- (not four-) hour shifts because exhibits couldn't be left. I was moved from the playground, which was not easily carried off, to the camping and boating exhibit, an exhibit that proved to foster marvelous conversations (more on these below) because we were outside, and people could relax as they

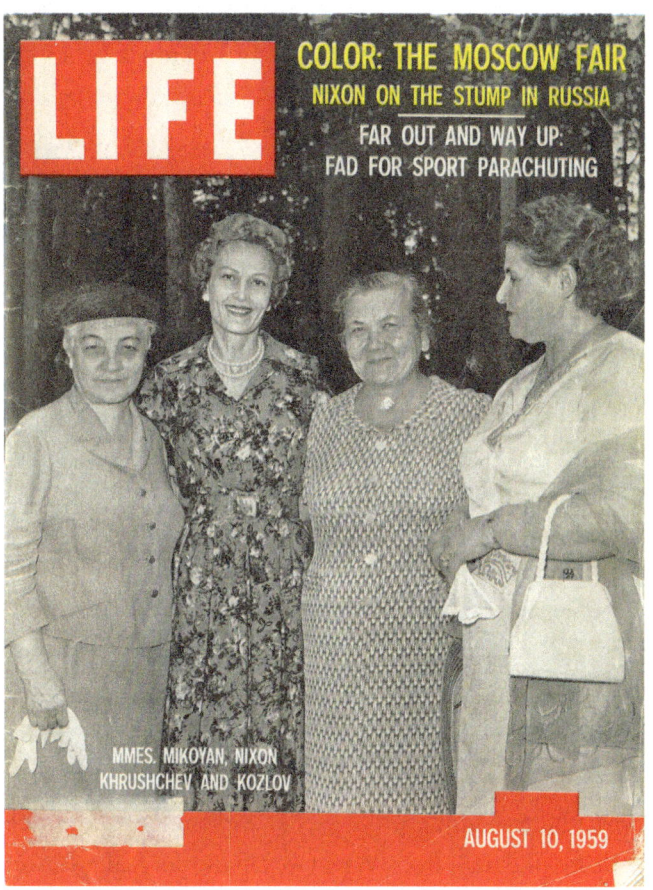

Politically Elite Attendees at the Opening Night of the Exhibition. From left to right: Madam Mikoyan, wife of the First Deputy Premiere of the USSR; Pat Nixon, wife of the Vice President of the United States, Nina Khrushchev, wife of the Premier of the USSR, and Madam Kozlov, wife of the Secretary of the Communist Party.

contemplated the beach wagon towing a pop-up trailer tent, a real lagoon with small sailboats and an exhibit of outboard motors. Next to the camping exhibit, in a grove of birch trees, was Gaston Lachaise's bronze *Standing Woman*, a voluptuous, naked, muscular woman. I was the closest guide to the statue, which was on loan from the New York Museum of Modern Art, and I regularly defended her, saying "of course, that was the way American women looked." The Soviets liked that answer.

The first two nights after the opening I was sleepless, my brain churning on how to meaningfully answer questions. Our fair was the first opportunity Russians had to find out about America from an American. It was a chance to compare what they had been taught in school, told at the factory, learned over the radio, and seen in movies to what we portrayed. Plus, the fair was entertaining; it had a model house where Khrushchev and Nixon had their famous debate, an operating beauty parlor where the guides got their hair done, rock and roll dance performances, a Circarama film showing the American countryside, a computer that could answer questions, color TV, modern art that was totally different from the socialist realism of Soviet art (Khrushchev said it looked like someone had pissed), free Pepsi-Cola, and guides, like me, answering questions about Americans and their lives. When we left the fairground at 10:00 p.m. a blocks-long line had already formed for the 11:00 a.m. opening the next morning. We were true entertainment, as well as education, and I worked to do my best to answer questions. It was exhausting, but exciting. I was running on adrenaline.

In my letters home I included a list of the questions we were being asked. These, verbatim from more than sixty years ago, included:

- Are the children of the unemployed starving?
- How much does a worker have to pay for his children to go to school?
- How much does it cost to go to college?
- Why don't women in America work; don't they resent being housewives?
- Why do Americans believe in God?
- What about segregation?
- Why has America surrounded us with military bases?
- Why don't you recognize Communist China?
- How could a worker buy this tent you have in your exhibit?
- You mean in America, people don't have to register when they move from city to city?
- Do you like the Soviet Union?
- Had your press distorted what you see here?
- Who are your favorite Russian novelists?
- Do Americans learn Russian?
- Are you afraid of us overtaking you?
- Would you like to stay here?
- Do you have a young man?
- Why don't you marry a Soviet?
- Will you be allowed to talk freely when you return to America?
- How many theaters does your city have?
- Does your city have an opera company?
- What percentage of the women in America have anesthesia when they give childbirth?
- What does your father do?

- You mean your family has three cars?
- How did your brother manage to find housing when he got married?

The Soviets were trying to find out about America, how Americans would answer about America, what America had done for its citizens. They seemed to be saying: "We live in a socialist system which is building Communism. Our state has given us many things and is giving us more. Look what the socialist system offers to the people of the future. What does your capitalist system offer? Don't you think that our system has given more to the worker?"

I talked about social security and the social safety net and America's work toward integration. I talked about how Americans, particularly my family, lived. Sometimes I would see a glint of understanding in someone's eyes. Other times someone would leave my exhibit with disbelief. Occasionally I would see someone come back to hear more about "my" America. As I walked in Moscow on my day off, Muscovites often recognized and talked to me and told me what they liked in the fair; other times they recognized me and denounced me and the fair.

A quarter of the citizens of the Soviet Union were killed or wounded in World War II. In the crowds at the fair, there was a dearth of the thirty- to sixty- year-old men who had been lost while holding and then advancing the Soviet military lines at whatever the cost. Those who had survived were building a new life for their children, building a new era, an era launched by Sputniks. Again and again, they told of how they knew what war was, of how they had eaten the dogs and cats. They had known war, terrible war. They supported their government, believed in their government. The average Soviet did not feel oppressed. Rather they felt that they, with their government and Khrushchev, were building a new future with peace and friendship.

In the excitement of finishing college and embarking on being a guide I had had little time to think about what life might be like in the Soviet Union. I recognized the Soviet Union for its military might and its highly functional T-34 tanks that had helped win World War II. I recognized it as the society that had launched the first satellites. I knew of its Olympic prowess. I also knew it was dedicated to a single party, Communism, that used prison camps for labor, and watchtowers and plowed borders to prevent its citizenry from leaving.

What I found in 1959 was a nation that had the support of its people, a nation that was building back from a devastating war. There was much that was not forced labor camps. Education and medicine were available for all. There were art museums, ballet troupes, concerts, folk performances, and a circus in which mice parachuted out of an airplane. There was an abundance of well-maintained parks. There were essentially no beggars and Nixon was publicly reprimanded when he threw coins to a crowd of onlookers. The streets were clean. There was good public transport, including the famed Moscow subway. It was safe to walk outside at night. The citizenry had social standards which they supported, telling me that I was not cultured should I cross my legs while sitting on the streetcar.

But the standard of living was astoundingly low and except for freshly baked potato bread (which was delicious), the goods for everyday life were just not there. Housing was as limited as the goods. People lived in apartments where multimember families lived in a single bed/sitting room and shared a communal bathroom and kitchen with two to three other families. If one wanted to live in another part of the city, one looked to trade (not buy) apartments. It was another world, another way of governance, another philosophy of life. It was a nation that had not included consumer goods or housing in its priorities. Rather it had prioritized defense, heavy industry, and sports and given its citizenry the goal of overtaking the United States.

As we were nearing the end of the exhibit, guides from the Russian exhibition in New York were returning to Moscow and appearing at the fair. These guides were the ultimate hecklers who combined facts, lies and opinion to champion the Soviet Union. A man approached me as I walked toward my exhibit. He asked me what I thought of Moscow, but instead of answering his question, I—realizing he was one of those dreaded returned guides—asked him how he had liked New York City. And then, a moment happened—looking into each other's eyes, we silently acknowledged the extraordinarily different worlds we had been part of that summer. I proceeded on to my exhibit. He went on to tour the fair. He had returned to his world, while I, in just a few days, would go back to my world.

The fair closed on September eighth. On the ninth, we flew to New York City where my parents met me at the airport. We visited my Russian teacher in her Brooklyn apartment where I got to say thank you. I had brought her *mishki* chocolates (a bear cub version of Hershey's kisses), not appreciating that they, reminding her of her youth, would bring tears to her eyes. And then, we drove home to Boston. I gave talks to the local churches, schools, rotary clubs, all of whom were fascinated to hear about the fair and my experiences in the Soviet Union.

Just as the Soviets knew very little of what life in America was like, Americans knew very little about life in the Soviet Union. In my talks I showed scenes of the fair combined with scenes of everyday life in Moscow.

I had received an opportunity which very few Americans at that time had: spending a summer behind the Iron Curtain addressing the questions of Soviet citizens about America. These conversations had given me a sense of the people behind the "smiling" Stalin of my high school social studies book. This Moscow chapter of my life temporarily closed while I obtained a master's degree in biochemistry, but reopened in 1961 for guiding at a traveling exhibition. In contrast to the 1959 exhibit, the 1961 exhibition took place during a freeze in Soviet-US relations. If Stalin had still been alive, he would have been frowning.

CHAPTER 4:

Master's Degree in Biochemistry, Return to Russia (1959–1962)

I returned to Boston just five days before undertaking my master's program in biochemistry at MIT. I had "discovered" science in my undergraduate years at Swarthmore and would now continue with that interest in graduate school. An apartment on Newbury Street had been leased by Marion Hale, a classmate from Swarthmore, who would be getting a master's in chemistry at Boston University. Our apartment, a one bedroom, was palatial by Moscow standards and easy walking distance to both MIT and Boston University.

I remember very little from that first year at MIT. I do remember purchasing a slide rule that would fit in my purse and buying used books in Harvard Square to try to understand chemical fugacity. I also remember what a male environment it was. There were very few ladies' rooms. In the Biology Department, which had more women than most courses, there were but a handful of female graduate students and no female faculty.

The first semester at a new school is often the hardest, and that was certainly true for me at MIT. Not only was my scientific coursework at Swarthmore less rigorous than that at MIT, but I was bone tired from my summer in Moscow. At the end of the first semester, three of my finals were scheduled in a row: morning, afternoon, morning. I did not have time to review my full notes for the third final—an important final—in biochemistry. I was sure that I had failed. When my grades came in, I heaved a sigh of relief, I had a C and no Ds. I assumed my C was in biochemistry, until my roommate pointed out to me that my A was in biochemistry and the C in physical chemistry. In retrospect, I think the only reason I survived that first semester at MIT was that my brain had been sharpened by my summer in Moscow, where I had been operating in Russian to both understand and respond to questions.

By the second year, I was more acclimatized. By this time, I was working on a thesis—a mundane project on thiamine phosphate phosphatases in yeast. The project was uninspired. However, it was clearly defined, and I rapidly finished my master's degree. Two years later, when I went on for a PhD, I was careful to go forward in a lab doing fundamental and exciting work.

At first my social life was fallow. There were lots of young men who pursued me, seriously pursued me, but none that caught my fancy. My social life blossomed when Wally, an MD who was taking courses at MIT as part of his hematology fellowship at Tufts Medical School, began to sit next to me. Our first date was spring skiing at Mount Snow, where I poled around the rocks as I followed him down the bunny slope. He wasn't dismayed at my lack of skill, giving me a kiss as I inched past a particularly formidable rock. When summer came, we sailed his Lightning class boat, the *Ondine*. The *Ondine* was fast, all sail, with windows in both the main and jib to be able to see and not run into whatever was to leeward. I manned the jib, wearing my Moscow dress-white cotton gloves to protect my hands. We sailed out of Marblehead where my parents kept the *Palometa*, a forty-two-foot motorsailer. The *Ondine* was much faster than the *Palometa*. We could, and did, sail circles around her. My parents became fond of Wally, including him in family events.

Although we never married, Wally would become the "lifelong" man of my life, the one man outside of my family whom I truly loved. It is hard to say why Wally and I came to care for each other as we did. He was fun, and very easy to talk to. We both liked outdoor activities. I respected his being an MD. He wasn't at all taken aback by my becoming an educated woman. We got along with each other's friends. And the chemistry was right, we liked sitting next to each other, being close. There was, however, an incompatibility in religion. Neither of us was active in our respective faiths, but he was Jewish whereas I was Protestant. My not being Jewish made a difference to his family and was a contributing reason for us never getting married.

As I was completing my master's program, I received a letter from the United States Information Agency asking if I would be interested in being a Russian-English speaking guide for "Transportation-USA," an exhibition that would open in Moscow and then travel to Stalingrad and Kharkov (the Russian name for Kharkiv) in Ukraine. The timing was perfect, and I accepted a second guiding job which would start in September 1961 and end in January 1962. I was still curious about the former Soviet Union and the traveling exhibition would give me the opportunity to travel there as well as in Europe on my way home. This time I would bring my winter clothes and ice skates. Wally and my parents would see me off from the observation deck at Boston's Logan Airport.

The traveling exhibit was a small exhibit, just eighteen guides, many of whom had worked, like me, at the much larger 1959 Moscow exhibition. Major exhibits were a Cessna aircraft and a Ford Thunderbird. I would be one of two guides who would show the Thunderbird. Our uniforms were Pan American and Trans World Airlines captains and stewardess uniforms. In contrast to 1959, when the United States and Russia enjoyed a relatively cordial relationship and many of my off-duty hours were spent with Soviets, by the fall of 1961, Russian-American relations were tense, and my off-duty time would be spent almost exclusively with other staff at the exhibition.

The Cold War tensions in 1961 arose from multiple factors. In May 1960, The Soviets had shot down a high-flying U-2 reconnaissance plane. The Americans claimed it was an off-course weather craft, only to have the pilot, Francis Gary Powers, who had parachuted to safety, acknowledge his intelligence collecting mission. Also, In January 1961, John F. Kennedy had been inaugurated as president. Our new president, America's youngest president, had neither the experience nor the relationship with the Soviets that our departing president, Dwight D. Eisenhower, had enjoyed. Ike's western front had worked with Stalin's eastern front to defeat Hitler's forces in Europe. In contrast, Cuban exiles, supported by Kennedy, had attempted an invasion at the Bay of Pigs on the Southern coast of Communist Cuba. In August 1961, the East Germans had started the construction of the Berlin Wall cutting off West Berlin from East Berlin and East Germany.

Both the Soviets and the Americans were testing and building nuclear arsenals.

Despite these aggressive interactions, the US-USSR exchange programs continued. However, in response to the burning of a Soviet flag at a Russian exhibition in Minneapolis, our exhibit was not allowed to open in Moscow, even with the exhibit being fully installed and the guides in place on our side and the anticipated hecklers (provocateurs) ready to go on their side.

The opening was reset for October 19th in Stalingrad, the second city of the tour. In the down time, the guides were given filing work to do at the Moscow embassy. Concerned about the weakness of my Russian language skills, I went to the Soviet Institute of Foreign Languages, where a director, after multiple phone calls, assigned me a marvelous teacher. My teacher, an older woman, helped me with answers to what I deemed would be frequently asked questions. Because Soviets had limited outfits, I wore the same clothes to all of our lessons. In her academic life she translated American poetry into Russian. When asked if there was something I might get her from the States, she expressed an interest in books of Sandberg's and Frost's poetry. I had my mother directly mail them to her. These books were but a small token of my immense gratitude to her for helping me with my Russian. And, she most likely had had an interesting time helping me, an American guide, work on answers to the social and lifestyle questions Soviets were most interested in. When the exhibit opened, I would have fewer hecklers than most of the guides. It may have been due to her debriefing her authorities (whom I am sure she had to report to on the Russian lessons) that I was a genuine student, not a provocateur trained by the US Central Intelligence Agency. It was also likely due to the Soviets being genuinely interested in the Thunderbird and its 20-liter V-8 engine, an engine which the engineer, who had been sent with the travelling Cessna, had explained to me. I could take off the air filter, test the oil level, and point out the spark plugs. Sounds simple, but it was fascinating to my audience.

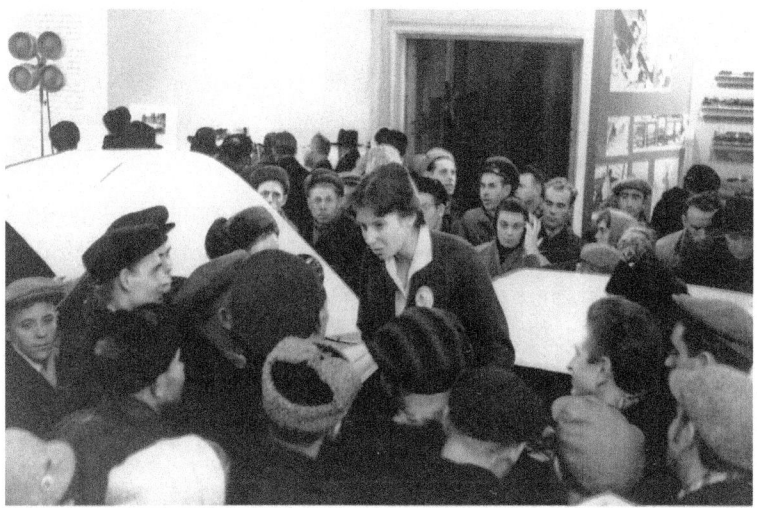

Exhibiting a Ford Thunderbird. I am in a TWA stewardess uniform. We worked without microphones, to have better control of the conversation.

On the second trip to Russia, we were followed everywhere we went. When each of us left the hotel, two Moskvitches (a Soviet car) with a driver and two passengers would pull out behind us. Having the "tails" was not all bad. They were personal positioning systems who knew the local environs, and once I had appreciated how to use them, could give good directions. I felt secure with them and instead of trying to shake my tail, always gave them time to board the subway I was about to board.

Once the embassy's scut work had been accomplished and the Moscow exhibit disassembled, we were given time off until we reported for work in Stalingrad. The guides had received two different types of visas to the Soviet Union. Most guides received visas limited to the cities where exhibits were to take place. But I, and one other guide, a male, had received our visas late, and been issued "all-union" visas. This meant we could go anywhere in the Soviet Union.

Given we had "all-union" visas, we chose an adventure, taking the Trans-Siberian Railway from Moscow to Irkutsk. We would spend six days on the train and have one full day in Irkutsk before we needed to return to duty in Stalingrad. Irkutsk lies on the shores of Lake Baikal, an enormous inland lake, three quarters of the way to Vladivostok, the eastern end of the Trans-Siberian Railway. There were three classes of travel: soft in compartments of four, hard in compartments of four, and hard in dormitory-style cars, where an entire car was fitted out with bunks, as seen in the movie *Dr. Zhivago*. We elected hard, in a compartment for four. The trip would end with an Aeroflot flight from Irkutsk to Moscow, a change of airports and then a flight to Stalingrad. We purchased our trip from Intourist, the pricey but mandatory Russian travel agency.

As for food, we provisioned ourselves with bread, a wheel of blue cheese and some grapefruit. Once en route, we found peasants peddling hot food in metal containers. We ate on the train, leaving the containers at the next station for return by a westbound train. There was a dining car on the train, although I do not recall our using it. Communal bathrooms with running cold water were at each end of the car. Freshening up did not include changing one's clothes. Each car was under the governance of a conductress who lived in a compartment at the end of the car. Among her duties was serving glasses of hot tea from a samovar. One paid for tea with sugar. Tea without sugar was free.

Our compartment mates were a middle-aged couple, who were travelling with a large bag of apples. They regularly sorted the apples to remove and eat any that were spoiling. They were good travelling companions. The train stopped briefly at small stations and for twenty minutes or longer at larger stations. To get to the other side of the tracks, passengers and luggage went under the train. Once we realized that this was how it was done, we, too, went under the train to investigate and shop both sides of the tracks.

In the Ural Mountains, we crossed from Europe to Asia, a crossing marked by a tall post with Europe engraved on the western side and Asia on the eastern side. The towns we were passing through reminded me of the lives of my grandparents. Horses and carts (or sleighs) were in use. Houses were wooden structures, except in cities where stucco was a favored building material. In mid-October, it was cold, and snow was accumulating. Most railroad crossings had a hut occupied by a woman who held up a ping-pong-paddle-sized stop sign for traffic while the train passed.

My favorite Siberian city was Novosibirsk. We arrived in Novosibirsk in the early evening with the train stopping long enough for us to walk into the city, one of the largest in the former Soviet Union. During World War II, the Soviets had moved much of their heavy manufacturing to Novosibirsk to protect their supply of weapons and munitions. After World War II, it made Novosibirsk its "Science City," a center for science research and education. Novosibirsk had an upbeat air with its mustard-yellow stucco buildings mellowed by gently falling snow and charmed by horses pulling sleighs.

Time on the train passed rapidly. Once the Soviets realized that there were Russian-speaking Americans onboard, we had a steady stream of visitors. Our Soviet compartment mate helped shoo the visitors along if the conversation started to become raucous or belligerent. Between stops, we looked out the windows and at stops we deboarded and negotiated with the peasants for food.

Irkutsk, itself, was an utterly charming village with sturdy, brightly painted wooden homes nestled on steeply rising lakeside hills. Its population, many of whom had Mongolian features, hunted, and fished. We luxuriated in multiple hot showers and ate from the Soviet menu that was the same across the entire Soviet Union. After my trans-Siberia experience, if I had needed to live in Russia, I would have headed to Irkutsk, away from the politics of Moscow, surrounded by nature and gourmet smoked fish.

On our return through Moscow, the Twenty-Second Congress of the Communist Party of the Soviet Union was in full swing. The city was festooned with Soviet flags and red stars to both welcome and dazzle its roughly 4,500 delegates. Communism was at a peak in popularity and Khrushchev, who had taken power after Stalin, presented the goal of completing the building of Communism in twenty years. The delegates voted to accept further de-Stalinization: Stalin's remains would be removed from the Lenin Mausoleum and cities named after Stalin, renamed. This renaming would include Stalingrad, our destination city.

Stalingrad is best known as the site of one of the bloodiest battles in the history of warfare with an estimated 1.2 million deaths. Both the Germans and the Soviets fought to hold positions no matter the cost The defeat of the Germans at Stalingrad in 1943 marked a turning point in World War II, which would end two years later in Victory in Europe Day. By 1961, despite the horrendous destruction, which included carpet bombing, Stalingrad had been rebuilt and was a pleasant riverside city. From our hotel, the Intourist, we could easily walk to the exhibit hall as well as to the esplanade along the Volga river to watch the river boats go in and out of the port. These boats carried agricultural goods and peasants, with peasants sleeping beside their goods in the river terminal.

The hotel Intourist, was on the central square of Stalingrad next to the hotel Stalingrad. The square, the size of a football field, was surrounded by loudspeakers that played music and gave the news. In the square was a prominent statue of Stalin. The exhibit had been running but a few days, when the morning movement of workers across the square halted as they listened to the message coming from the speakers—Stalingrad was to be renamed. Once the announcement finished, movement in the square resumed. By that evening, Stalin's statue had been removed and at the hotel next to us, the word "Stalin of Stalingrad" had been removed from its neon lights. Several days later, the city was renamed Volgograd and "Volgo" appeared in the place of Stalin on the renamed hotel. At the exhibit, my audience would chortle when they asked me how I liked Stalingrad; and I would reply that I quite liked Volgograd.

The exhibit was open a mere twenty-one days before we dismantled it to proceed to our final city, Kharkiv. Kharkiv, the second largest city in Ukraine, did not have the charm of the Volga River and its marvelous esplanade. We celebrated Christmas in a room adjacent to an exuberant wedding where the bride and groom kissed each time glasses were clanged. In my letters home, I was counting the days until I would fly out of Moscow.

By New Year's, I was back in Moscow where the marines guarding the embassy needed to look at my documents, to appreciate that I was an American. Living on Soviet food for three months, which included essentially no vegetables, I had lost some of my natural facial color and my clothes were getting run-down. My haircut was a Soviet haircut. I greeted 1962 in Red Square, which was empty except for our small group of Americans and a small group of Soviets with a costumed Saint Nick. On New Year's Day, one of the embassy marines took me skating on the frozen paths of Gorky Park. The Soviets, fabulously good skaters, had strap-on metal runners for skates. I skated to piped-in music and passed by hot cocoa stands. It was a wonderful last outing in Moscow. The next day, I left the Soviet Union to fly to Vienna. When the pilot announced we had entered Western airspace, the passengers spontaneously erupted in applause.

Vienna was the first stop on my homeward-bound travels. It would take several weeks before I would not be checking for my tail. Walking in downtown Vienna, a policeman jumped out of his traffic booth to reprimand me for an inappropriate street crossing. The reprimand bounced right off me; I was so glad to be out from behind the Iron Curtain, not so much for the lack of greyness, but for the relief from repression that had come with being constantly tailed, constantly watched, and constantly challenged on this second trip.

I started my travels across Europe on the Orient Express.

First stop, skiing in Austria at Saint Anton. The two guides, a married couple with whom I was traveling, were also novice skiers. Although late in the day, we rented skis and headed up the lifts only to find ourselves on slopes way over our heads. We ended up taking off our skis and carrying them down the empty slopes as the lights of Saint Anton twinkled up at us. The next day we hired Ferdl, a rather stern instructor, who worked full days with us for two weeks. Ferdl, despite having described us to his fellow instructors as *alles ist schlecht* ("all are bad") when we began our lessons, paraded us in graceful loops down the mountain by the end, flaunting his prowess.

I reboarded the Orient Express with a new pair of skis and a custom-made burnt orange pair of slacks. The next stops were two weeks in Paris and a visit to Berlin with my mother. In Paris, my mother and I had a wonderful time visiting museums, attending concerts, and going to the Folies Bergère. We shopped for clothes, buying me a belted suede coat and a custom-made suit. I got my hair cut at a French beauty salon.

A visit to Berlin was orchestrated for us by the Wolters, the family of a German exchange student who had lived with us when my brother Tom was the one remaining child at home. We flew into Tempelhof, the airport that had been used by the Berlin airlift to provision West Berlin when the Soviet authorities had halted land traffic to the city. We could have travelled to Berlin by train, but I did not want to risk being on the ground behind the Iron Curtain where Soviet authorities might be idiosyncratic—especially toward someone whose passport indicated a prolonged period as an American in Russia. Flying would only subject me to American passport checks. Hermann's cousin, a student in Berlin, met our flight and showed us around. My memory of 1962 West Berlin is open spaces, cleared of rubble but not rebuilt because of the uncertain future of the city.

The last stop on my European trip was a visit to Jan in Edinburgh. I took British Rail, which in contrast to the Orient Express assured me that single women were automatically placed in all-female cabins. Jan was a newlywed living in a small flat.

Arriving back in the United States, it was Wally this time, not my parents, who would meet my plane in New York. I first spotted him on the balcony overlooking the arrivals hall. He first recognized me by my walk, which he said was tentative. It took time to get through customs where the officer challenged the price of my skis—my one item that had its full price on the bill of sale. I finally convinced the official that I had spent only $59 on the simple wooden skis. And then I was in Wally's arms and Wally's car, sitting next to him on its pre-front-wheel-drive bench seat, catching up with him as we headed north to Boston and dinner at my parents' home.

After leaving the Soviet Union in 1962, I would not return, or use my Russian again, until 2007 when I was a scientific speaker at a symposium in Saint Petersburg on the status of human immunodeficiency virus (HIV) vaccine research. My talk, given in English, entitled "DNA/MVA Vaccine for HIV/AIDS," was well received. Saint Petersburg in 2007 was a different world from the Soviet Union that I had experienced in 1959 and 1962. People were fashionably dressed and in the upscale area of Saint Petersburg where we were staying, it was easier to find sushi than borscht. But when you took the subway, as I did, it took you back to a more Soviet world where one did not cross one's legs when seated.

CHAPTER 5:

PhD Research on Messenger RNA (1962–1965)

Once home, I visited the MIT Biology Department to check in with my classmates and look for a job. My classmates informed me that a new lab, the Darnell lab, was helping build molecular biology at MIT, bringing the study of animal cells and viruses to MIT. Wearing my Parisian belted suede coat, I approached Darnell and secured a position as a technician. In contrast to the research in the lab where I had obtained my master's degree, the research in the Darnell lab was exciting, addressing how cells with the same DNA came to possess different functions. At MIT, technicians were allowed to take a course at no cost. I still looked at my future life as that of a homemaker who had been temporarily involved in science. This was the path that my mother, who had a master's degree in chemistry, had taken. But I couldn't resist enrolling in my allotted course and soon was not only participating in the course but sitting in the front row at departmental seminars. My interest in molecular biology had crept up on me. It was a new field, an exciting field opening insights into how cells grow and differentiate into the many functions of living organisms. I had found my professional field.

Life was good except that I was in my highly marriageable years and Wally was not proposing. In my naivete I had not been concerned that Wally was Jewish. He had been born in Berlin where his father, a successful physician, was a medical professor. With the rise of Hitler and anti-Semitism his family feared for their lives and in 1934, as restrictions on the ability of Jewish people to hold jobs were put in place, they had emigrated to America. His father found a job as a pathologist in Batavia, a small town in upstate New York. Wally and his younger brother, Michael, helped their parents with the English language and American customs. The local synagogue became a mainstay of their life.

In Judaism, Jewish identity is passed through the woman. This meant that, according to Jewish tradition, Wally could not have Jewish children without marrying a Jewish woman. For Wally, despite loving me, marrying a non-Jew was too big a break with his family.

I cannot remember what precipitated the breakup, but it happened over the 1963 Christmas holidays. Devastated, I decided to reenter graduate school, becoming a candidate for a PhD in Darnell's lab. The qualifying exam, which was administered once a year, would take place just two weeks after my reentry. While we were walking to cash checks at the MIT bursar, Sheldon Penman, a Bell Labs physicist who had joined the Darnell lab to learn molecular biology, opined that any concept in biology could be mastered in two weeks. I decided to take the exam, telling the skeptical Darnell that, if

I failed, the department rules were that I could have a second chance. My devastation over the breakup with Wally was drowned out by hard work as I spent the next two weeks at my desk. Much to everyone's amazement, I not only passed but did better than expected.

My having done well in the qualifying exam more than met the Department of Biology's expectations for a PhD candidate. The minor in chemistry, which at MIT involved a remarkable amount of math, challenged my very modest training in mathematics. Looking back, I wish I had taken more courses in mathematics, including statistics, because of the importance of mathematics to quantitative science. In contrast to the chemistry minor, I breezed through the foreign language requirement, taking the exams in Russian and French. I was on my way to a PhD.

The house full of young women in Central Square where I had been living had ended with graduations and marriage. Supplementing my stipend with the substantial nest egg I had earned in Russia, I moved into 100 Memorial Drive (a modern, high-rise apartment building within the MIT campus), hired a cleaning lady and purposefully limited work to nine to five. One does not usually hire a cleaning lady when one goes to graduate school. Also, a typical graduate school student does not limit work to eight-hour days. By doing both, I acknowledged that I was entering a man's field but was still committed to being a mother and homemaker. If I could not use household help and manage my graduate work in eight-hour days, I would not have the time for that hoped-for family and be able to compete with my male counterparts, who, if they were typical academics, would be working at least ten-hour days.

My thesis research addressed a central dilemma of biology: how does DNA, which is the same in all cells of an organism, produce the different types of cells that constitute the organism? In 1963 when I initiated my thesis, the dogma was that different regions of DNA produced RNAs in different cell types. The RNA that a cell expressed, termed messenger RNA (mRNA), then determined what proteins the cell made and the cell's structure and function. In other words, the DNA that was the same in brain and muscle cells would express (produce) brain-specific mRNAs in brain and muscle-specific mRNAs in muscle. For my thesis, I worked on the size of mRNAs and the time it took for newly synthesized mRNA to move from the nuclear DNA where it was synthesized to the protein synthesis machinery in the cytoplasm of the cell. My studies showed that newly synthesized mRNA had a broad range of lengths and that it moved within minutes from the DNA in the nucleus, where it was synthesized to the cytoplasm, where at its earliest appearance, it was already associated with polysomes, the structures that synthesize protein. My peers were interested in my research, attending my lab seminars, discussing it in the hall, and explaining it to their spouses and significant others.

Midway through my thesis research, Darnell was recruited to Harry Eagle's newly formed Department of Cell Biology at the Albert Einstein College of Medicine in the Bronx. Fortunately, I had sufficiently fulfilled my degree requirements that I could move with Darnell to complete my thesis work at the Einstein and still graduate from MIT.

At the Einstein, as at MIT, there was the excitement of discovery. Eagle instituted a rule that no questions could be asked until a seminar speaker was at least fifteen minutes into their

PhD Research on Messenger RNA

presentation. As I look back on my graduate education, I realize that MIT provided me with a highly quantitative approach to research whereas the Einstein immersed me in the early thought leaders in cell and molecular biology. At both institutions, our in-house seminars were ahead of our outside speakers.

While at the Einstein, I lived on West Sixty-Ninth Street, in the first block off Central Park. It was a studio walk-up with a landlady who entertained herself by keeping track of the comings and goings of her renters. West Sixty-Ninth Street was a wonderful location, central enough to be easily able to walk to the major museums, Broadway, and Greenwich Village. I became a member of the Museum of Modern Art, where I visited Lachaise's naked, bronze woman that I had verbally defended at the American Exhibition in Moscow. Aunt Barbie, who liked to spend the fall in Greenwich Village, came for her annual visit to the city. We spent time together, attending a showing of Uncle Howard's collages, riding the Staten Island Ferry, and eating at her favorite restaurants.

But perhaps most important, while still in Cambridge, Wally, a man whom I really cared about, had reappeared as a suitor. Despite the breakup, we still enjoyed each other's company. He, proud of my PhD thesis work, helped me with the move to New York City and regularly spent weekends in New York. It was a vibrant, wonderful year.

In June 1965, Darnell returned with me to MIT for my thesis defense. The defense, a success, was followed by toasts at the faculty club. I drove Darnell to the airport and then joined my family and Wally for champagne and an evening sail on the Palometa in Boston Harbor. As painful as the breakup with Wally had been, he had provided the impetus for me to get something that very few women at that time had—a PhD from MIT. He had opened the door for me to have a career in science. But at the same time, by failing to seal our relationship in marriage, he had opened the door for me to blossom in my career, to grow into a larger world of which he would be a smaller part.

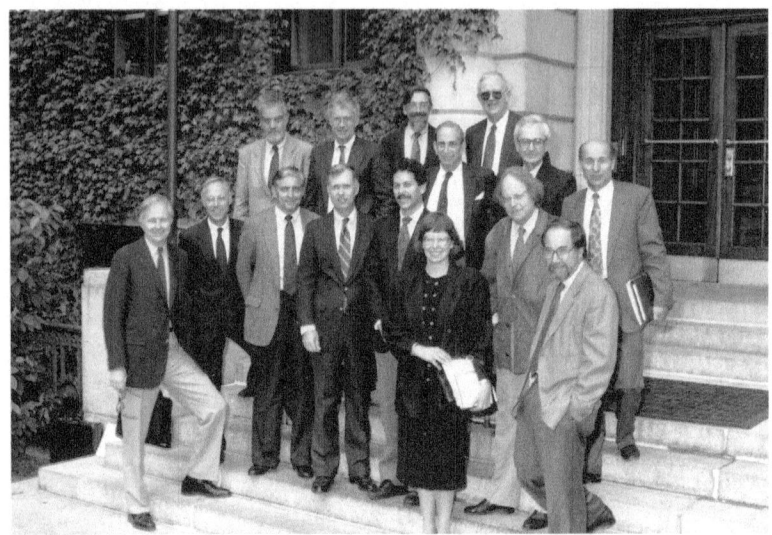

Jim Darnell and His Early Trainees in Molecular Biology. We are celebrating Darnell's 60th birthday. Darnell is front, left. I am the one woman in the picture and am standing to the left of David Baltimore, who stands far right. The birthday celebration took place in 2000 at Darnell's then institute, Rockefeller University. In 2002, Darnell would be honored for his work on gene expression with the National Medal of Science.

CHAPTER 6:

Postdoctoral Training, and Marriage (1965-1967)

I had completed my degree in just over two years and instead of feeling ground down by the PhD process, I was exhilarated by the excitement of discovery and by my empowerment to study mRNA through molecular biology. I was looking forward to the next step, postdoctoral training. For my postdoctoral training I chose Harry Rubin's laboratory at the University of California Berkely. Rubin's lab specialized in work with the Rous sarcoma virus, a virus that causes cancer.

Rous sarcoma virus is named after Peyton Rous, who in 1911 identified a tumor in a chicken that he could transplant from chicken to chicken. First, he used small pieces of the tumor for the transplants. He next tested whether homogenates of the tumors, prepared by blending diced tumor with saline, could transplant the tumor. When the homogenates still caused tumors, he passed the homogenates through a filter with pore sizes that could pass viruses, but not the much larger bacteria. When the filtrates (solutions that came through the filter) caused tumors, it suggested that a very small agent, potentially a virus, was causing the cancer. He named this agent Rous sarcoma virus. In 1965, when I received my PhD, Rous sarcoma virus had just been shown to contain RNA (not DNA) as its genetic information. If an RNA virus could cause a tumor, the information (message) for that tumor must reside in its RNA. By working with a tumor causing virus, I should be able to gain insight into genes that cause cancer.

I wrote to Rubin, only to receive a response that he did not have room, but there was a young professor down the hall who might have room. He mentioned that he was going to be in New York for a meeting. I responded that I was interested in his lab (not the lab of the young professor down the hall, whom I ended up marrying) and set up a time to meet him while he was in New York City. At the end of the meeting, Rubin offered me a slot for a July 1, 1965 start in his lab. He had actually had room in his lab all along and had been hedging his bets to get someone truly interested in his lab by testing how I would respond to his suggestion of taking a position in another lab down the hall. I accepted on the spot and applied for and was awarded a two-year National Science Foundation postdoctoral fellowship. I was on a roll!

Although Wally had reappeared and I was still fond of him, I had been burned once and did not trust that he would ever marry me. In addition to his being Jewish, there was something about his psyche and his life experience that precluded him from finding a solution to marrying a non-Jewish girl and taking on the responsibility of marriage. Returning to Boston as Wally's perpetual girlfriend did not seem a realistic route to a family. And, I not only had the opportunity to work in a field in which I had relevant experience (the new field of mRNA) and which could have solidly important outcomes (identification of genes that can cause cancer), but I also loved California from my college summers as a counselor at Camp Timberloft.

I advertised for a person to drive across the country with me and found a young British woman, a nascent hippie, who had made it to the United States and could not wait to get to San Francisco. My cross-country drives during college to work at Timberloft were before the Eisenhower interstates were built and had taken me through the American countryside at a relatively slow pace. This time we barreled across the United States on the new interstates with only one real stop, in Taos, New Mexico, to visit Aunt Barbie.

On arriving in Berkeley, I stayed with a friend from MIT until I secured an apartment. Within a week of my moving into my apartment, my car was broadsided by a uninsured young motorist who had not obeyed a stop sign. In the collision, my head jerked sideways and was gashed by hitting the open driver's window. The police took me to the emergency room, where the gash was stitched up. The first person to come to my aid was the young professor from down the hall from Rubin's lab. He arrived at my apartment with an ice cream cone and then started taking me out to dinner. It turned out that he, Bill Robinson, was an MD whose interest in infectious disease had led him to do research at the Berkeley Virus Laboratory.

The organization of the Rubin lab turned out to be casual to say the least. I was not assigned a lab bench or desk space. Taking it upon myself, I sat at the empty desk where there was no window glare, only to be told by Ruthie, a long-standing tech, that I couldn't sit there, Hanafusa had sat there. Hidesaburo Hanafusa is one of the greats in tumor virology. I was a young female with a gashed head, apparently not worthy of occupying the spot. Not yielding to Ruthie, I stuck to my guns and kept the seat. As my work progressed, I even did honor to the seat, extending findings that Hanafusa and his wife had made.

In the Rubin lab, I learned how to culture animal cells and showed that cells, transformed by a specific strain of Rous sarcoma virus, the Bryan strain, were producing noninfectious virus particles. These noninfectious particles were later shown to contain viral RNA that included the *src* (sarcoma) gene of normal chicken cells. The *src* gene would represent the first identified cellular gene that, if inappropriately expressed, could cause cancer.

Meanwhile, Bill Robinson (the young professor down the hall), who had come to my rescue when I first arrived, was busy courting me and had realized that he was regularly taking to dinner someone who, like himself, liked to hike. Our first major hike was Mount Whitney, at 14,505 feet, the highest peak in the contiguous United States. Instead of taking the classic Mount Whitney Trail (21.2 miles round trip), we headed for the north face, a shorter, steeper climb. It turned out that the last ascent by the north face trail was cliffs embedded in scree (scrambled rock) and snow. We turned back to have time to make it down before dark. Despite not having summited, it was a spectacular hike. We would later reach the summit, taking the classic trail.

Bill was attracted to me, and unlike Wally, it was not long before he proposed. We enjoyed each other's company, both liked the outdoors, and both wanted children. In contrast to Wally, there were no religious problems. Neither of us were active churchgoers, but we both had Christian heritages, his grandfather had been the pastor of the First Methodist Church in Jackson, Mississippi. I cried when I accepted Bill's proposal.

It meant that I would not marry Wally. I was attracted to Bill, but it was not the same as my earlier attraction to Wally. I also had dated Bill long enough to know that he could be bossy and self-centered, but I was young and felt I could get along with him.

I called to let Wally know that I had accepted a proposal from Bill. His reaction was that he was going to kill Bill, and he got on a plane. This behavior was totally outside the norm for Wally. I let the airlines know that a distraught suitor was on his way and a representative from the airlines and I met Wally at the gate when he landed. There, it was obvious that he had come with his shaving kit, but no weapons. The airline representative took us to a room where we could talk and booked Wally on the next flight, the red-eye, back to Boston. There was not much I could say, or he could say, to change the situation of my being committed to Bill. After Wally left, I called his best friend, who met him when he arrived in Boston.

The wedding was at Christmas In my family home with only the two families and the minister present. I found a simple white dress with a leopard skin belt. Without its belt, it was quite suitable for a wedding. A friend lent me a piece of lace for the veil. At the time of the marriage, Massachusetts required that the license be obtained a week before the marriage. A lawyer put the paperwork in place so that Bill could marry me using a license that had been obtained the day before the marriage. To do this we had to go to the property court. Both the lawyer and my father apologized that my marriage was making me property. The licensing officer, an older woman, was disapproving until she realized that I was not marrying my father, but a young suitor who was flying in. Bill flew in and picked up the wrong bag, which he discovered when he could not unlock it.

The correct bag was located, and bags exchanged. The next day I went with Bill to meet his family who flew in from Indiana. We took them to the then new John Hancock building, where they stayed in the penthouse. The rehearsal dinner took place on the observatory floor. The families met each other against spectacular views of Boston.

The wedding was a seven-minute Protestant ceremony. My father walked me downstairs to meet Bill and his brother Dave, who had entered from the kitchen. The service was officiated by Reverend MacIntosh, our longtime family minister. Appropriate entry and exit music were played on a new hi-fi my parents had acquired for the occasion. After the ceremony, there was a reception in the dining room. We were toasted with champagne. We cut the cake and fed each other cake. The mood was family-oriented, with my nieces and nephews having fun with their new uncle. A photographer from Bradford Bachrach took pictures; the candid shots show a radiant bride and groom.

We left immediately after the champagne for a honeymoon that started with a weekend in New York City. I called Darnell, who asked me what my new last name was, and held a small gathering for us in his home. We then flew to Santa Fe to visit Aunt Barbie and Uncle Howard and to ski at the new Taos resort. There, we slept on the floor of the art studio of a friend of Aunt Barbie and were wonderfully hosted on Christmas Day by Aunt Barbie and Uncle Howard. While there, we visited the galleries and bought Howard's oil portrait, *Young Indian*. As a wedding present, Howard gave us a charcoal, *Procession*. Howard and Barbie had taken us to the real procession, the carrying of a statue of Mary and the baby Jesus around the central common area of the pueblo on Christmas eve. As the procession passed, men fired rifles into the air and boys threw pieces of stone into fires that lit the procession. The bits of stone splintered into pieces as they exploded from the heat. Howard's charcoal captured the darkness of the procession we had witnessed.

It had been a simple but happy wedding for a marriage that unfortunately would falter with time. However, it was a marriage that would bring me (and Bill) the blessing of three wonderful sons. In contrast to becoming a wife, becoming a PhD from MIT did not falter, but rather provided me the foundations for a career I loved in which I used molecular biology and chickens to study the genetic basis of cancer and pioneered the use of DNA as a new method of vaccination.

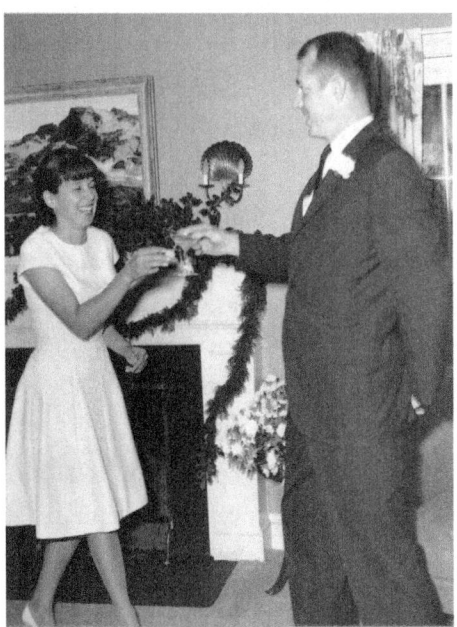

A Christmas wedding. The groom passing a celebratory glass of champagne to his bride. The wedding was in my parents' living room.

CHAPTER 7:

Early Marriage Years and Time Out for a Family (1967–1975)

My major memory of my early days of marriage was being tired. I had hired a cleaning lady, and we went out to dinner several times a week, but I was carrying groceries, which now included beer for Bill, up three stories and just learning to cook. As soon as food was on the table, Bill would wolf it down. By the time I had my plate served and sat down to eat, he would be done and have the TV going. I came from a family where one waited for everyone to be served to eat and where one enjoyed conversing during dinner. I learned to eat faster, but never got over the TV jarring normal conversation.

    Bill also liked to go out. The dishes would be left in the sink for me to wash later. It never occurred to him that he could and should help. He only needed six hours of sleep whereas I needed eight to nine hours. He tried to train me to need less sleep. I successfully objected to this but was not successful in getting him to assume more of the responsibility for the groceries and meals. We did hike and go to the opera in San Francisco. We also socialized with other faculty at Berkeley. It was not all bad and I was committed to the marriage.

In the fall of 1966, on our return from an international virology meeting in Tokyo, we agreed that I would stop taking birth control pills. By this time, Bill was being recruited by Tom Merigan to join the Division of Infectious Diseases at Stanford Medical School. Merigan was building a faculty who could use the power of new molecular techniques to improve health care for viral and bacterial infections. Bill accepted and we started looking for a house in Palo Alto.

Our move date was accelerated by the Vietnam War. The Gulf of Tonkin Resolution had authorized the then US president, Lyndon B. Johnson, to take any measures he believed necessary to win the war and the ground war had expanded to close to 400,000 troops. These troops needed doctors. Doctors who taught medicine were considered essential and not at risk for being drafted. Doctors who were not teaching medicine were fair game for the draft. Bill's summons arrived in the summer of 1967. Stanford immediately went to bat for the essential nature of his work, instructing him not to report. Meanwhile, we had become expectant parents, and my due date was the third week of September. We were to close on a Palo Alto house on August 30. Movers were scheduled for the thirty-first.

Our first born, Billy, however, did not wait for the third week of September, and arrived in the midst of the move on August 30. Bill dug out the obstetrics book, which had been packed, to see if what was happening was really happening, and we drove for Stanford where my obstetrician came in from vacation to do the delivery. The obstetrics staff, settling in for a typical first labor, came to check me, only to realize that Billy was making his entrance. There was a rush for the delivery room for the arrival of a wonderful, lusty-lunged six-pound, one ounce baby boy. In 1967, the practice was to not have babies stay in the mother's room. At feeding time, a loudspeaker would announce: "Babies are coming, babies are coming, will all mothers please wash their hands." And then, I would wash my hands and get to hold him, feed him, and love him.

Bill rescheduled the move for September first and finished the packing. We had planned to get baby gear once in Palo Alto. The only gear we had was a baby buggy passed on to us by another fellow in the Rubin lab and a baby scale, given to me by my tech, who knew I would be interested in weighing my baby. Bill shopped for layettes, diapers (still cloth) and a washing machine and dryer. Billy and I stayed in the hospital for three days, at which time we came home to a house full of boxes. The milkman, the first to realize that there was a new baby in the house, left a very helpful baby book. Bill started work at Stanford on September 5, the day after Labor Day. I was overwhelmed and called my mother for help. She had been in Nantucket, sailing with my father. She immediately flew west.

I knew nothing about babies and did not wash my hair for three weeks after Billy's arrival so that I could hear him, should he need me. It took a few days to get him gaining weight. I nursed lying down because it was easier for him to latch on. At the first postnatal visit, our pediatrician, an exceptionally effective doctor, had me start rice cereal as a thin gruel. The rice cereal helped both with weight gain and the timing of feedings, which I was doing on demand, roughly every two hours.

Happily, things began to fall into place. The new washer and dryer were installed. My mother got more baby clothes, bought groceries, and took over running the sprinklers to water the lawn. Bill was becoming settled at Stanford. We were getting up and running. I washed my hair and began to relax. I read an article at this time which said there are four major stressors in life: deaths, births, moves, and new jobs. We had experienced three of these four all at once! But we survived and a new baby is a wonder. Both Bill and I watched for the first smile, which was not long in coming.

After Billy's birth, Bill and I consciously set out to have a condensed timeline for our family. I wanted to be home with the children but still have the potential for a career in science. Having a cluster of babies would allow me to take time off to be with the babies, toddlers, and preschoolers and still have years for more full-time work after they were in school. Given this plan, Al arrived thirteen months after Bill; and Tom arrived thirteen months after Al. My life was full-time babies and toddlers. When Tom was a newborn, he was feeding eight times a day (on demand), Al was eating four times a day, and Billy was on his father's schedule of three times a day. I never had more than two in diapers as I toilet trained Billy before Al arrived, but I did run a load of wash every day. I nursed Billy and Al for three months and Tom until he was weaned to a cup. When I was nursing, the boys nursed our cat, Kitty, or a stuffed animal.

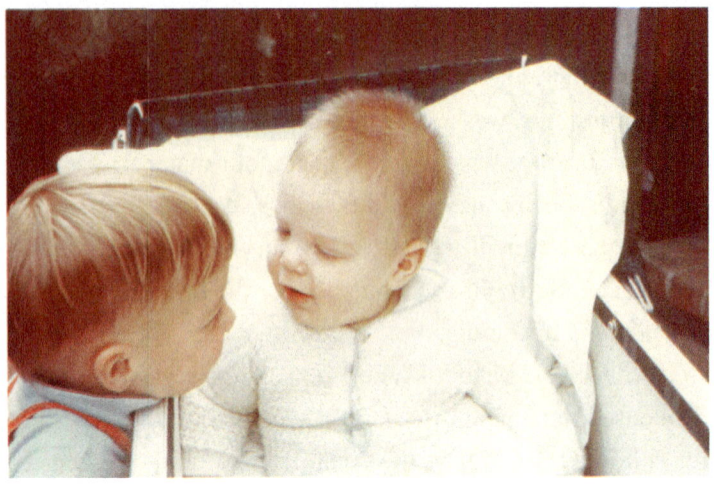

Billy Interacting with Al. Al is in the baby buggy. When Tom arrived, the two older boys incorporated him into their activities. The three boys provided each other with hours of entertainment.

We had a routine. After we got up in the morning, I would start the wash and then load Billy and then Billy and Al, and then Al and Tom and then only Tom into the baby buggy to go to a neighborhood park. Graduates from the baby buggy rode plastic motorcycles and then, when big enough, big wheels to the park. The boys would swing, climb on the equipment, and play in the sand until noon when we would head home for lunch. After lunch, everyone, including me, would take a nap. When we woke, the boys played, and I did housework. The older boys automatically included the infant, who was frequently in the Jolly Jumper—a type of hanging bouncer that is no longer considered safe for babies. When the youngest got to where he could do pull toys, they all three pulled toys up and down our long hall.

If there was a fight, I would put whatever they were fighting over on top of the refrigerator and all three of them into their beds. Their beds were all in one room and their stuffed Snoopy dogs, which had good ballistic as well as comforting qualities, were soon flying and the boys happily interacting. At the final bedtime for the day, Bill and I would read to them —*Pat the Bunny* for the infant, *Curious George* and Richard Scarry's picture books for the toddler, and *Babar, Little Toot,* and *The Little Engine That Could* for the preschooler. As for getting up in the morning, we had a Mickey Mouse clock with 7:00 a.m. marked with tape. When the hands of the clock reached the tape, Billy, who was the first to be able to turn a doorknob, would open the door and the three little boys would roll out in moist dydees to join me and Bill in bed.

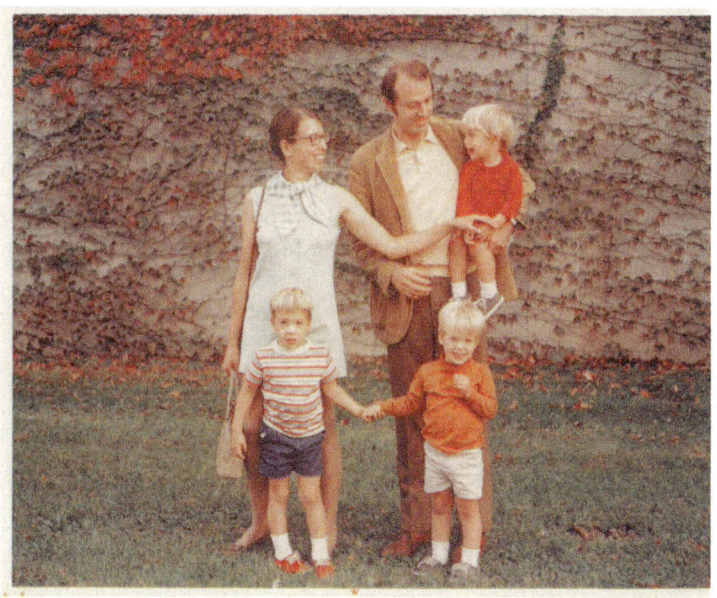

The Robinson Family. This picture was taken by my mother-in-law, Aline Robinson during our 1970 trip to visit family. We are in front of a wall of ivy at Indiana University where she was Dean of Freshman Admissions and my father-in-law, Sid Robinson, was a Professor of Physiology. Billy and I are on the left while Bill, holding Tom, and Al are on the right.

As the boys turned four years old, we started them in Ruth Woods Nursery School, two or three mornings a week. I would work in Bill's lab, helping with the routine culture of chicken cells from embryonated eggs on the mornings they were at nursery school and be home by the time they were home for lunch. Cell culture involves only a few hours of work changing culture dishes and feeding with liquid medium followed by several days in which the cells grow. It is an appropriate job for someone who, like me, had but a few hours in the lab before returning to the continuously remarkable growth and development of the boys.

Ruth Woods, who headed the nursery school, pointed out that Billy was inappropriately using a d in many of his words. For example, "Kitty" was "Ditty," and "swimming" was "swimding." I got a language book out of the library and began to practice words with Billy every day before nap. We would catch Kitty (who didn't particularly like language practice) and sit on Billy's bed practicing. I learned to do mostly words Billy could correctly pronounce with only a few hard ones, typically polysyllabic, sprinkled in. Our pediatrician, who was monitoring the language issue, was impressed and asked me what we had done. I answered, "practice." Language practice, although simple, had been fun for Billy because of Kitty and his success with the easy words, which, when possible, I strung into colorful versions of his and his brothers' activities such as "Tom and Kitty went swimming with a duck." They also were fun for me because we made progress.

During these years when the boys were preschoolers, Bill was focused on his Stanford career. He was home for dinner and worked only part-time on weekends. In the evenings, he watched sports. I typically preceded him to bed. He liked to run, and on weekends we would all go to the Stanford track where the boys played with the equipment while he ran. He also liked to go to the movies, and I found babysitters so that we could go out. Disappointingly he was far from a helpmate—very different from my father and brothers. Life was easier when he was travelling and I did not have him as well as the boys to care for. I totally had not appreciated that he could be so enthusiastic about having children, but so uninvolved in their raising. When Billy portrayed his family in a first-grade drawing, his teacher commented on the hierarchy. The largest figure, whom she had assumed would be his father, was Al. I was also large and Tom of intermediate size. Bill, the smallest, reflected his father's minimal involvement in their early lives.

Our neighborhood, in "old Palo Alto" was a mature neighborhood without many children. However, at the park, we found other children; two of the mothers, Joan Hancock and Ellen Nachtrieb, became lifelong friends. Across the street, we became friends with Mr. Davenport, a retired salesman, who used two canes to walk. Mr. Davenport, who had no children of his own, had a special place in his heart for the boys. He included them in the conversation and noticed and praised their accomplishments. One evening, when Mrs. Davenport invited me to a piano concert, he babysat the boys, who could not wait to tell me how they had fooled Mr. Davenport by sleeping in the wrong beds. Another friend was Emil, who drove a fruit and vegetable truck. Emil would stop to show his wares and chat while he restocked our produce. Many families grow up without active fathers. I had not planned to be such a family, but there is life without a true helpmate and Bill was advancing at Stanford and providing a salary.

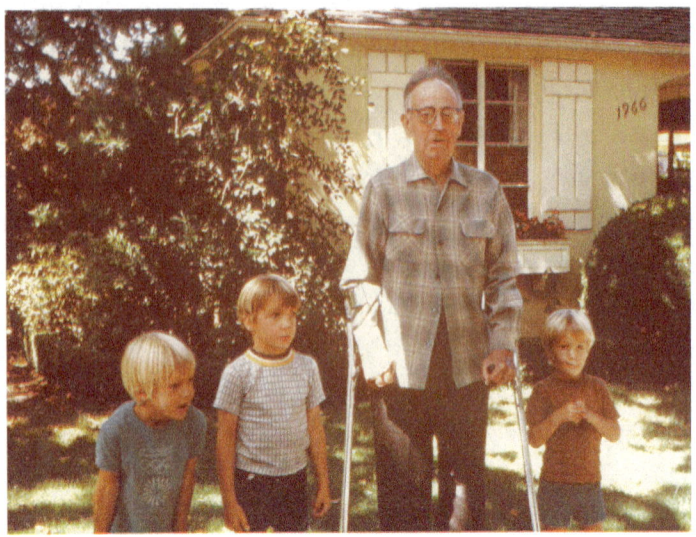

The Boys in a Serious Discussion with Mr. Davenport. From left to right: Al, Bill, Mr. Davenport (a favorite neighbor), and Tom. The boys and Mr. Davenport were great conversationalists. He had been a salesman and knew how to bring them out.

By 1974, Bill had worked seven years at Stanford and was eligible for a sabbatical, which he wanted to take in London. Billy was in second grade, Allen in first grade, and Tom in kindergarten. I was working two to three hours in the mornings to be home by the time Tom was home from kindergarten. Bill found a sponsor at the University College in London where he could broaden his background in immunology. Bill's first choice had been for both of us to work in Robin Weiss's lab at the London Institute of Cancer Research. Since Weiss did not have room for both of us, I wrote to see if he might have room for just me, part-time, with my own salary. Weiss was a thought leader in tumor virology and had just co-written a broadly read book, *RNA Tumor Viruses*. I was extremely pleased when Weiss responded that he had space for me. At the Weiss lab I worked too few hours to have my own project, but I did become friends with the other fellows with whom I shared a cheek-by-jowl office. These new colleagues included several future leaders in the field of tumor virology. On the practical side, I learned how to freeze viable chicken cells—something that would prove important to my future work and something we had not succeeded in doing at Stanford.

The plan was for a six-month sabbatical. We found a fourth floor walk-up in the Belsize Park region of London and looked for a school. A church-sponsored school turned out to have room for the boys. Bill would walk the boys to school in the morning, I would pick them up at the end of the school day. The British schools were different from primary schools in Palo Alto. Instead of working with massive pieces of paper, students did art in a student booklet. After each drawing, the teacher would ask the child what it was, and then write the word under the picture. The boys would then copy the word under the teacher's word. The British had a series of books for beginning readers describing the adventures of an ant, a bee, and a kind dog. The boys loved the series. Al and Tom learned to read in London, while Billy solidified what he had learned in first grade in Palo Alto. Once a week, the school went swimming. Each child folded their clothes into a neat pile. When they first went to the beach on returning to the United States, my sister-in-law could not get over the neatly folded piles of clothes. They did class trips such as riding on a canal boat. In keeping with the school being a church school, the boys would pray for good weather before the trips.

We regularly went on weekend outings. The boy's favorite was the Hard Rock Café where they could eat American hamburgers. Of the trips outside of London, Stonehenge was the big hit. In 1974, visitors could still clamber on the giant rocks. My favorite trip was Greenwich, which one reached by a Thames riverboat. The Royal Observatory designed by Christopher Wren was at Greenwich. It was at this observatory that Greenwich mean time, long the world standard, was established. Bill senior liked going to the theater. We took the whole family to see *Jesus Christ, Superstar*. Bill and I also went to experimental theater, where a play I could have done without featured a secret code tattooed on the private part of the male villain. To retrieve the code, the villain had to have an erection.

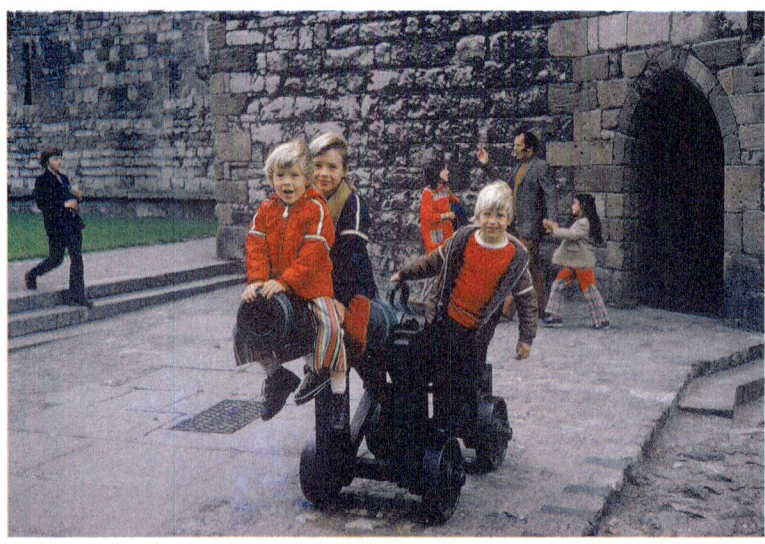

The Boys Playing on a Cannon at Greenwich. Al is hanging off to the right, Tom is in front, and Billy is in the middle.

Our other activity was climbing mountains. In Scotland, Bill and Billy made the top of Ben Nevis. The challenge was cold-foggy weather, not the altitude. I played with Al and Tom at the bottom. In Wales, we all made the top of Mount Snowden, with me and three exhausted boys coming down on the cog railway. On a European trip, we waited at the Matterhorn for four days for the weather to clear. Each day, Bill and a boy would hike to the Hörnli Hut (10,700 feet), a favored launching point. After all three boys had been to the Hörnli Hut, we gave up and proceeded to Mont Blanc. At Mont Blanc, the weather was promising, and Bill managed to secure a guide. The guide knew almost no English outside of "Yosemite." The night before the ascent, Bill and the guide slept at a base camp, partway up Mont Blanc. They hiked early, starting at 3:00 a.m., to minimize the chance of thawing snow placing them at risk for avalanches. The boys and I played at the bed and breakfast, which had an outdoor ping-pong table and where my high school French was our means of communication.

We ended up coming home a month early. Although our income was much higher than that of a typical London family, our London rental fee was more than we were receiving for our Palo Alto home, and with no car or washing machine, we were living way below our Palo Alto standard of living. Home early, we house-sat, taking care of Thor, the homeowner's German shepherd, while we waited for the lease on our house to be up.

We were all happy to be back in Palo Alto. The boys, pleased to be home, were able to start school on time with their classmates. I had the luxuries of a car and American appliances supporting my daily life. While the London immunology lab had not caught Bill's interest, I had found my hours at the London Institute of Cancer Research productive and had established new and valuable personal connections in the field of tumor virology.

CHAPTER 8:

Return to Work (1975)

When we came back from sabbatical, the boys were in first, second, and third grade. The time had come for me to return to a more active life in science. The plan was for me to work 75 percent time, from 9:00 to 3:00, to be able to get the boys off to school and then be home soon after they got home. In preparation for my working 75 percent time, I found Mrs. Vlaming who could drive the boys and do errands, tasks which Espaze Guillory, our pre-London childcare help could not do. Mrs. Vlaming was also punctual whereas Espaze, who relied on her children to give her rides, had always been plus or minus an hour.

When I returned to work, it was in Bill's laboratory where my task was to oversee the supply of chicken cells to be used to study Rous sarcoma virus. Rous sarcoma virus is a replication-defective virus that requires helper functions for its growth. These helper functions were first discovered as infectious viruses called Rous helper virus (or Rous associated virus). With time it was appreciated that uninfected chicken cells also could provide help to Rous sarcoma virus. This second form of help was called chick-helper-factor. What Bill needed was chicken cells that were not only free of infectious helper virus but also free of chick-helper-factor. Chick-helper-factor was an enigma. What was it? Why did different embryos have different patterns of chick-helper-factor? And most importantly, how did these patterns relate to the ability of Rous sarcoma and its associated helper viruses to cause tumors?

To make sense of what I was observing, I needed to keep track of the pedigrees of the embryos I was characterizing for chick-helper-factor. Bill called Dr. Lamoreux, the lead scientist at Kimber Farms, the breeder that supplied our eggs, to set up a meeting. When I arrived at the farm, Dr. Lamoreux took a double take—he had not expected a female Dr. Robinson, wife of the male Dr. Robinson. Despite my being a woman, he was interested in further developing the lines of chickens that Kimber had developed for high egg production. Initially, I cultured cells from pinfeathers to type the roosters and hens producing the eggs I was typing. To get pinfeathers, Kimber Farm's staff pulled mature feathers and then two weeks later harvested the regenerating feathers. The pinfeathers were then sent from Fremont, California, where Kimber Farms was located, to downtown Palo Alto on the Greyhound Bus.

Our studies showed that the lines of chickens had different patterns of chick-helper-factor. Working with Dr. Lamoureux we set up a breeding program to enrich for the different patterns of expression. I made use of what I had learned about freezing viable chicken cells while on the London sabbatical to preserve cells with the different patterns of chick-helper-factor.

Unexpectedly, Kimber Farms was acquired by DeKalb Ag Research. I drove out to Kimber Farms to meet DeKalb management, who had decided to move the Kimber chicken lines to Illinois. I was welcome to have the sublines I was working on; but there would be no support from DeKalb for maintaining or further developing the sublines. If I could not find money to support the chickens at Stanford, my chicken breeding program, and studies on how chick-helper-factor affected cancer induction by Rous sarcoma and its helper viruses, would be over. I turned to Robert Huebner who had secured a large federal contract ($60 million) to study the role of viruses in cancer. Huebner, a staff member at the National Institutes of Health (NIH) in Bethesda, dispatched a colleague to check out my program. Based on the colleague's recommendation, Huebner agreed to award me a $10,000 subcontract to support a chicken caretaker and chicken feed for one year. This support, the first recognition of my work on chick-helper-factor, was modest, but adequate for what I needed.

Bearing data on chick-helper-factor, I next went to Stanford Lab Animal Medicine to obtain space for the chickens. Despite the interest of chick-helper-factor to cancer programs at the National Cancer Institute, Stanford Lab Animal Medicine was not interested in housing chickens with defined patterns of chick-helper-factor. I then went to Tom Merigan, who headed the Division of Infectious Diseases and was Bill's boss. Merigan, recognizing the importance of defined patterns of chick-helper-factor for Bill's research funding, arranged for us to visit Lab Animal Medicine together. We walked in and Merigan and the director of Lab Animal Medicine slapped each other on the back and animatedly discussed the upcoming football game between University of California, Berkeley and Stanford. At the end of the exchange, which had nothing to do with chick-helper-factor, chickens, or cancer, Merigan and the director again slapped each other on the back. As we rode the escalator up from Lab Animal Medicine, which was in the basement, Merigan said "well Harriet, you have your chickens." Though dumb struck by how things had been done, I was elated to have my chickens.

My assigned chicken space, about a thousand square feet, was a roofed, open-air shed with chicken wire "walls" located across the medical school parking lot behind the old anatomy building. I now had to prepare this space for receiving and caring for the chickens. Concerned that chicken cages were being taken for breeding illegal fighting cocks, Kimber Farms happily donated chicken cages to Stanford for studies on cancer induction, a highly legal activity. Stanford engineering hung the donated cages in rows separated by four-foot wide aisles and hooked up the water system (each cage had a waterer that the chickens pecked to activate). Droppings would fall on the concrete floor. Using a wooden form, I poured a six-inch high cement barrier along the chicken wire wall separating my chicken area from an adjacent area occupied by caged monkeys. The cement barrier worked quite well at preventing water from the chickens running into the monkey area, or water from the monkey area running into the chicken area. For determining the pedigrees of chicks, Kimber Farms donated stacked brooders with wire boxes (the size of shoe boxes) for hatching and wing banding clutches from the same parents. They also provided me with feed bins, shovels, brooms, hoses, rubber boots, and even a glass-sided incubator that had been used at Easter to hatch chicks for local schools. Using my Huebner subcontract, I hired a part-time chicken caretaker and bought chicken feed.

In preparation for the transfer of my chickens to Stanford, I revisited Kimber Farms. Dr. Lamoreux showed me the Farm's breeding area, which was still in operation. By some cages, there were warning signs, "mean rooster." We sat down in the lab area where he counseled me on breeding chickens and encouraged me to use random breeding within sublines to maintain vigor. He then showed me how to do artificial insemination and had me practice collecting semen (fortunately from non-mean roosters) and inseminating hens (who can also be mean—especially when they sense you do not know what you are doing). Once I had the hang of what I was doing, it proved to be a simple procedure with neither the roosters minding donating semen nor the hens minding receiving the donated semen.

All in all, about seventy singly housed chickens were transferred to Stanford for studies on how chick-helper-factor affected the induction of cancer by Rous sarcoma virus. With time, I added chickens representing chicken lines developed at the US Regional Poultry Research Laboratory in East Lansing, Michigan. Working with my lines and the Regional Poultry Research lines, my colleagues and I would demonstrate that chickens had at least seven different patterns for chick-helper-factor. Our unravelling the presence of chick-helper-factor, although tedious, turned out to be immensely important, laying the foundations for seminal studies on viral-induced cancers.

The sabbatical had been both physically and psychologically hard on me. It was physically hard to keep house in London and psychologically hard to not have friends who could provide emotional support, which was certainly not coming from my husband. When I got back to Palo Alto, I was run-down. Bill complained that I was out of shape—needed to exercise. He wanted more variety in the dinner menu, but when I cooked something new, he would object that he did not want to eat whatever it was that I had cooked. It was frustrating.

Working in Bill's lab, although part of the master plan, was decidedly the wrong thing to have been doing. It meant that all day, as well as all night, I was subject to his domineering attitude and lack of empathy. When he came stomping in the door at night, headed for the toilet, the boys and I would recede into ourselves. At breakfast, I would serve his English muffin and peanut butter in the dining room while the rest of us gathered around the kitchen table. He was growing apart from us, and we from him.

On returning from sabbatical, the lab needed a secretary and Bill hired Phyllis, a recent college graduate who had just arrived in the Bay Area from the East Coast. Like Bill, Phyllis was a runner. He began coaching Phyllis on her running. Phyllis and he compared running diaries and then began to run together. He began inviting Phyllis to dinner, not every night but often enough that I became uncomfortable. Phyllis was gaining weight while I was losing weight. Things came to a head when Bill invited Phyllis to accompany us to the medical virology meeting at the Keystone Resort in the Rocky Mountains. When we arrived, late in the day, the boys and I were deposited in our condo while Bill and Phyllis went out to dinner.

The meeting featured morning and evening sessions, giving the participants time to ski in the afternoon. The boys were enrolled in day care at the ski school. Bill, Phyllis, and I set out on cross-country skis to explore the old mine roads that laced through the woods. In no time, they were far ahead of me, out of sight. I stopped to rest in a deserted mining cabin.

Bill found me there, but I wanted nothing to do with him. I had had enough. I skied out to the shuttle bus stop and took the resort bus back to the lodge. I found a ride to Denver, called my parents, and flew home to Boston where my father, worried, met my plane.

For the next few days, I talked with my parents while recovering from an ear infection. My mother did not like Bill. She had seen how inconsiderate he could be while she was helping with the babies. My father was concerned that I would not be able to raise the boys without a male presence, especially in their teen years. But I did not want to continue living with Bill. He had been an interesting partner, interested in the arts as well as medicine and outdoor activities, but also a negative partner. Meanwhile, Bill had made his decision, moving into a local motel, and emptying our safe-deposit box before I returned.

On my return to San Francisco, Bill and the boys met me at the airport and took me home, where the boys and I started our lives as a single-parent family. I took off my wedding ring. We did marriage counseling, which only brought out how estranged we were. The counselor pointed out that we never looked at each other and called each other Dad and Mother, our jobs in the family, not Bill and Harriet, our given names. Bill's family hoped we would get back together. I let the boys' teachers know what was happening. My brother Tom, who lived in San Francisco, began visiting us weekly. Tom also took the boys skiing. I could not understand how anyone could leave their children. But at the same time, it was like being let out of a cage to no longer live with Bill.

Despite the trauma of the split, I began to relax as the boys and I undertook life without Bill. I had always believed that the only way I would get to live without Bill was to outlive him. Now, I had been freed. Neighbors and friends commented on how good I looked. Our pediatrician asked a friend of mine what was going on because I looked so relaxed and happy, unlike the typical newly separated mother with young children.

It was an amicable separation, better than the marriage. We did not fight and did not snipe at each other. The boys, who had friends with divorced parents, accepted separation as part of life. The divorce lawyers and legal agreements did not come into play until a year later when the boys and I were leaving Palo Alto; the actual divorce occurred a further year later, well after we had moved onto our new life in Massachusetts.

During the separation, I continued to work in Bill's lab while I looked for a permanent job. My chicken lines were my unique ticket in the cancer research community. In addition to looking for job possibilities at Stanford, and through Darnell, my thesis advisor, and Rubin, my postdoctoral mentor, I responded to job postings in *Science* magazine. I was particularly interested in jobs close to family, in California or Massachusetts, but applied to positions all over the country. My applications consisted of a cover letter, a curriculum vitae, and a list of my major research goals. Rejections flowed back. It was discouraging. But I did not give up on getting an independent job. I did not want a job like most senior women in science had at that time, supporting someone else's lab.

Then, unrelated to my job search, an invitation arrived for me to speak on chick-helper-factor at Huebner's Annual Meeting on Cancer Viruses in Hershey, Pennsylvania. Since I was going to be travelling to the East Coast, I wrote to the recruiters for the two positions in Massachusetts. Both institutions—Clark University in Worcester and the Worcester Foundation for Experimental Biology in Shrewsbury, a suburb of Worcester—accepted my offer to visit. The Worcester Foundation emphasized that I could visit but that they would not pay my travel expenses. This was not a problem because my travel would largely be covered by Huebner for my speaking in Hershey and because I could stay with my parents and use my mother's car in Massachusetts. Mrs. Vlaming would stay with the boys in Palo Alto for the week I would be gone.

I spoke at Hershey and then proceeded home to Boston for the two talks in Worcester. The interview for the position at Clark University, primarily a teaching job, would be first. After my seminar, in a group interview, the faculty, who were baffled by chick-helper-factor, quizzed me on my willingness to move to Massachusetts. They took me to empty rooms that might become chicken rooms. On the way to a fast-food dinner, they showed me Worcester neighborhoods where faculty lived. I drove home to Boston, where my parents were waiting up for me, and reported on the job, which was far from what I was hoping for. I then washed my interview blouse to be ready for the Worcester Foundation on the next day.

The Worcester Foundation's main claim to fame is that it was the institution where the birth control pill was developed. The "pill," which is still used by millions of women, received US Food and Drug Administration (FDA) approval in 1960. By 1976, the Foundation had expanded into cancer research. In contrast to the Clark University position, the Worcester Foundation position was a research job. After my seminar, the director enthusiastically showed me empty lab space that was being built out in a new research building. There was plenty of room for chickens on the multi-acre grounds. A recruitment dinner was held at the very nice and regionally appropriate 1790 Restaurant and Tavern.

At the end of the dinner, I was verbally offered the job with the promise of an offer letter to follow. It turned out that the Foundation needed me not only to staff their cancer center but also because I was a woman. They had had a legal case over salary with a woman scientist. Before moving on, she had picketed the grounds with women pushing baby carriages. Hiring me would not only help their cancer center but represent their commitment to women scientists. I also needed them. I needed a research job where I could relocate the chickens. Ideally, I wanted a job that would be close to either East or West Coast family.

After dinner, instead of driving east for Boston, I drove west, back to the Foundation, to see if anyone was working at night. The lights were out. This meant the Foundation would not expect me to work at night. I could be competitive working nine to five and be home for supper and after supper activities with the boys. I would accept the Worcester Foundation offer and withdraw my application for a job at Clark.

The move was now on in earnest. During the summer and fall of 1976, I returned to the Worcester Foundation for several short visits to work on plans for my lab and the chickens and to find a house. (The boys remained on the West Coast with Mrs. Vlaming in charge.) I designed lab space into my office so that I would have an additional bench. The chickens would move after my move, as fertile eggs. I designed my chicken space to include a large room, which would house banks of cages, a food storage room with access from the outside as well as the inside, an incubator room for hatching chicks and a small lab. The facility was entered through a dressing room, where the staff would gown-up to keep the chickens free from infections. Waste went out through a waste room that had both outside and inside doors.

As for finding a house, it was December, a time when housing sales are low. There were a mere three possibilities in Shrewsbury, where the Worcester Foundation was located. I chose the one with boys similar in age to my boys, playing basketball in the driveway. My boys were excited because it had an above ground swimming pool. It was convenient, within easy biking, and even walking, distance of the Foundation, Spring Street Elementary School, and the town library. Money for the closing of the Massachusetts house came from my portion of the closing of the Palo Alto house. Money for travel for me and the boys and moving expenses for the family, the frozen cells, and the chickens, came from the Worcester Foundation.

My parents had come to Palo Alto for our last Christmas in California. They took our houseplants with them when they returned to Massachusetts. The moving van loaded our household goods and then drove to Stanford to pick up the frozen cells, which were in liquid nitrogen tanks. The movers treated the boys by letting them ride to Stanford in the sleeping area of the van. Bill then drove us to the airport where Uncle Tom as well as Bill saw us off. We had our ski gear with us and were headed for Utah where we would spend several days skiing with friends while en route to Massachusetts.

From Utah, the boys went on to Indianapolis to spend a week with the grandparents Robinson while I returned to California for the closing of our house, and to pick up Kitty and the frozen virus stocks and cells. I silently wept when my flight from Salt Lake City to San Francisco taxied past Frontier and Western airlines with the Wasatch mountains in the background. I was leaving the West and the promise of my now failed marriage behind.

While waiting for our car to arrive in Massachusetts, Uncle Dave, who lived in nearby Harvard, Massachusetts, offered us the use of his VW van. Uncle Dave, an astronomer, was seeing if his van could "drive" to the moon, 270,000 miles. The odometer, on its third cycle, was at about 20,000 miles, or a total of 220,000 miles when we were driving it. My Stanford chicken caretaker and his girlfriend, on their first leg of an around-the-world trip, would drive the station wagon from Palo Alto to Worcester. When it arrived, we would christen it with the license plate: "Hey Mom." I would keep this plate until Tom, my youngest, graduated from high school.

I had written to the boys' new school, Spring Street Elementary, that we were coming. The school welcomed the boys, with their classmates telling them where the pet store was. Billy's fourth grade teacher learned that we were reading *The Hobbit* at home, and read *The Hobbit* to Billy's class, making him extra welcome.

Shrewsbury, Massachusetts would be a very different place to live than Palo Alto. Palo Alto is home to Stanford, a premier institution of higher learning. Near San Francisco, it had the excitement of the early days of Silicon Valley coupled with a hippie vibe. Shrewsbury is a suburb to Worcester, a city of blue-collar workers that was losing manufacturing jobs. Its most novel feature was Spag's, a sprawling, heavily discounted retailer that only took cash. Spag's (without bags) sold everything in a unique jumble of product display: jelly jars next to automobile tires, udder balm next to razor blades.

At the time of the move, in early January 1977, we had been separated from Bill for a year, and the boys had become used to living apart from their father. At our last visit, in December, our Palo Alto pediatrician advised me to delay my start of work for a month so that I could focus on the transition for the boys. This was exceptionally sound advice, which I followed.

CHAPTER 9:

Balancing the Lab and Family as a Single Parent (1977–1987)

Immediate, happy events for the boys on our midwinter 1977 arrival in Massachusetts were the start of our Sunday night dinners with my brother Dave's family, who lived nearby in the town of Harvard. Uncle Dave and Aunt Ginger had five boys, overlapping in age with my three. The first weekend in Massachusetts, Uncle Dave took my boys shopping for hockey equipment, and we had the first of what would become weekly Sunday night dinners with Uncle Dave, Aunt Ginger, Jimmy, Peter, Andy, Jon, and Win. In the winter, the boys and Uncle Dave would play team hockey at the local ice-skating rink and Aunt Ginger and I would chat and make pies. In the summer, the boys and Uncle Dave would play baseball on a large field that they had mowed, and Aunt Ginger and I would enjoy each other's company as we picked berries and made jelly. Everyone looked forward to Sunday afternoon and dinner at the cousins'. This family tradition was followed until the boys were in high school and needed to tend to their homework. We were lucky

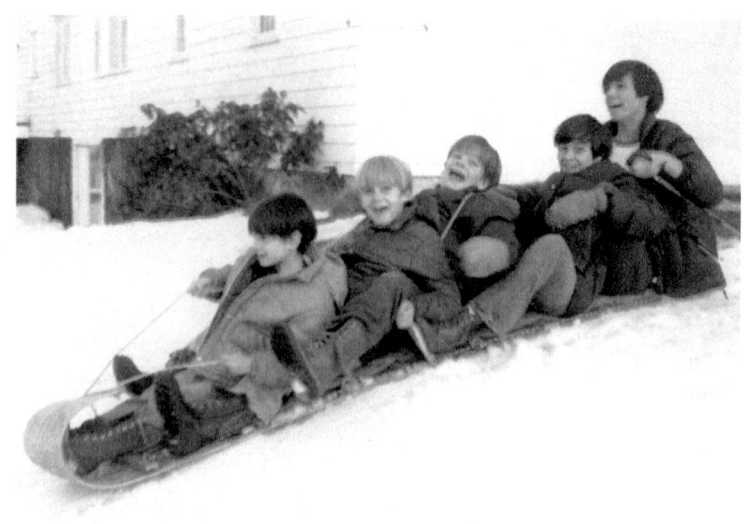

The Cousins. A happy feature of Massachusetts was spending Sunday afternoon and having Sunday dinner with the cousins. From front to back (youngest to oldest): Win, Jon, Andy, Peter, and Jimmy.

to be in Massachusetts and close to not only family, but an interesting and supportive family.

Immediately on arrival in Shrewsbury, I advertised for household help. It took several rounds to find a suitable person. The solution, Eunice, arrived pushing the garage door opener instead of the doorbell. She would become our "Mary Poppins" who would cook and be there for the boys until all three were in high school. In her twenties, she was the youngest of a large, politically active Worcester family. When there was a snowstorm, Eunice would arrive at work on a city snowplow. She was interested in the boys' activities and soon knew and ran the entire neighborhood. One of my favorite memories of Eunice is passing her and the boys on my way home from work. I was on my bike. Eunice was driving the car. The dog was hanging out the front passenger window and the three boys were in the back seat wearing their hockey helmets. Everyone, including the dog, was grinning from ear to ear. Later that evening I asked the boys why they had their helmets on—"Eunice drives fast" was the chorused response. When Eunice came back after the summer vacation, the dog would be so excited he would lose his cookies (upchuck). Driving fast or not, Eunice was a presence. We were very fortunate to have her. After we graduated from her care, she successfully passed the GED exam for a high school diploma and married a state policeman. The boys took on cleaning the house and running the wash because they thought that Eunice had been totally overpaid for what she did.

The boys readily adapted to the structured education at Shrewsbury Spring Street School. In Palo Alto, children roamed the classroom and had substantial freedom in their choice of learning activities. At Spring Street, desks were fixed, and the class taught as a group. The boys learned in both scenarios and were easily at grade level in both reading and math. Except for one teacher, who could not keep order, the Massachusetts teachers were very good, with Mr. Large being particularly supportive of Al, having him stay after school to help prepare class projects. After an altercation in the playground over a ball in which Al was threatened with being beaten up and had hot-footed it home in the middle of the day, we decided that when in the playground, he should stay in the vicinity of Mr. Large, which worked.

Our Shrewsbury home had only three bedrooms and there were five of us: the three boys, Eunice, and me. When we first moved, the boys all bunked in the room that was the master bedroom. We unstacked the double-decker bed so that they each had a freestanding bed. The boys slept in the sleeping bags that we had bought in Great Britain, a tie to their former lives. Eunice and I slept in the two children's bedrooms. Our first project for the house was to remodel so that everyone would have their own bedroom. We did this by adding doors to convert the first floor study and the living room into bedrooms. Bill and Al would move into the upstairs children's bedrooms, Tom would move to the living room bedroom, I would move to the master bedroom, and Eunice would move to the study bedroom. After these moves, the boys somehow considered Massachusetts home as they, without anything being said by me, switched from their sleeping bags to regular bedding. Tom kept the ping-pong table in his bedroom and set up a fish tank. Al built a narrow-gauge model train set into his bedroom. Bill had a telescope in his bedroom. The rooms were finished off by adding desks purchased for $25 each from the used equipment at the Worcester Foundation.

An unexpected plus for our Shrewsbury life was the return of Wally. At the time I purchased our Shrewsbury home, I needed a lawyer. I went to the Stanford library (this was pre-internet) and looked up the number of Herb, a lawyer who had been one of the gentlemen friends of the Central Square house where I had lived with a group of women while getting my master's degree. Herb readily agreed to help, and then, without telling me, called Wally, who had never married, saying, "Guess who is coming back to town." Wally's response was to invite me and the boys for Presidents' Day weekend to his recently acquired Vermont farm. The farm was near a local ski area, and we brought our skis. I slept in the loft with the boys. It was a wonderful weekend. After that Wally regularly came to dinner on Thursday nights. He was a great raconteur and the boys liked both telling him stories and listening to his stories. Wally and I no longer had a romantic relationship, but I had provided him with a family, a family that he came to love and that came to love him. He provided us with a loving male companion, who delighted in our conversation and activities. We were his "best show in town." Both he and my brothers became important male role models for the boys.

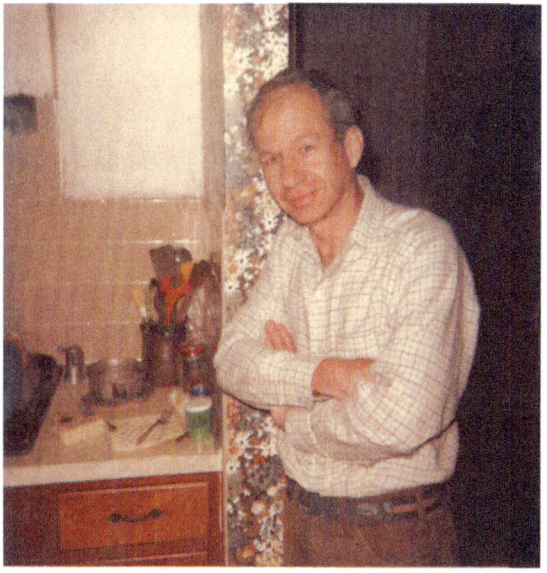

Wally. Walter J.K. Tannenberg MD, in our Shrewsbury home. Wally was beloved by both the boys and me.

The boys all did Worcester youth hockey, all played town soccer, and all participated in Little League. The hockey coach appreciated the boys because, even though they started as beginner skaters, they knew where they should be and were good scorers. Each year town soccer started just as the boys returned from the August visit to their father. We solved the problem of finding appropriately sized soccer shoes by buying one pair of each size to get the sizes we would need before they were sold out. All sizes ended up being worn. The Shrewsbury school system had an active music program. Bill took up the trumpet, Al the saxophone, and Tom the French horn and drums. They liked their respective instruments and occasionally accompanied Wally, who would play the piano.

The boys' father would stop and visit the boys when he came east for reviewing grants for the NIH or to give lectures. I would leave the house and stay at a friend's so that he could have the luxury of a home for his visit. Bill would not always let me know he was coming. One night, we were all in bed when just before midnight, the doorbell rang. The dog and I lifted our heads and hearing nothing, I tucked back under the covers. The doorbell rang again. This time, the dog and I got up and looked out the window and there was Bill. I let him in and gave him sheets and blankets for the hide-a-bed. In the summer, the boys would spend the month of August with their father in California. Once they were in high school, they had three-week winter and spring breaks during which they could visit their father. In the first years, the transitions back and forth were hard. When the boys were sad because they missed him, we would all sleep together in my bed.

Their father and I maintained a cordial but distant relationship. He and Phyllis married and divorced. Eventually he formed a lasting relationship with KeTing, a Chinese molecular biologist and entrepreneur. He and KeTing would marry and have a daughter, Sophie, whom the boys enjoy.

Camp Kabeyun, a boy's summer camp on Lake Winnipesaukee in New Hampshire, came to play an important role in the boys' lives. Kabeyun was run by my oldest brother, Nick. When they reached nine years old, the boys became campers for the July session. Once fifteen, they became counselors in training and then counselors. As young boys, they improved their swimming skills, eventually swimming to Ship Island. They learned to row, canoe, sail, and water-ski. Rock climbing and backpacking were popular as they became teens. Tom placed first in the camp tennis tournament. Wonderful clay figures and model boats came from the pottery and wood shop activities.

In their junior high years, the boys helped Uncle Nick set up camp. They worked for pay, getting the frogs out of the water lines, painting, sanding, setting up the waterfront, cabins, and departments, whatever needed to be done. As counselors, they would head both the sailing and trips departments. I would join the activities on weekends to cook for the pre-camp staff.

But the value of going to camp wasn't just the skills they gained at Kabeyun, it was also the friends they made, many of whom were sons of campers that my brothers had known when they had been Kabeyun campers. Once, when I was visiting, I went with Al for evening dock duty, a time when boys could informally take out the various watercraft. I soon realized that campers had come to the dock, not to boat, but to chat with Al as the sun went down.

Uncle Nick was a highly effective camp director, providing a culture that kept order while allowing his staff and campers remarkable freedom and responsibility. Years later, he would succumb to Parkinson's disease. As he failed, and lost his ability to walk and talk, a steady stream of Kabeyun alumni, including my sons, drove to rural Groveland, Massachusetts, where his family was caring for him, to visit and pay tribute to him.

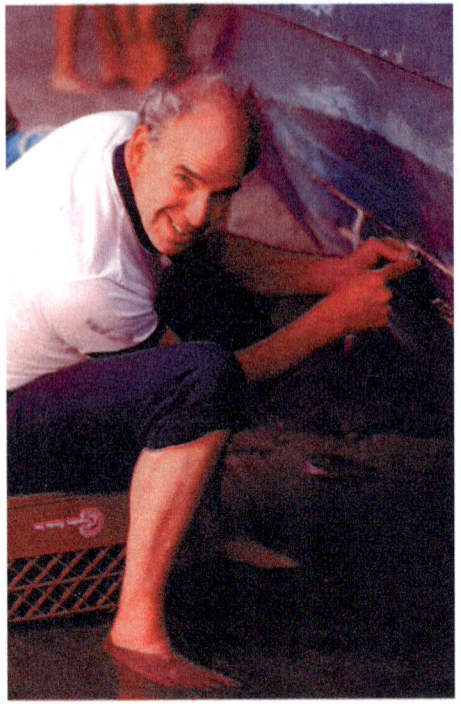

Uncle Nick. Uncle Nick in his element at Kabeyun, repairing a boat.

As a single parent family, we met with some discrimination in Shrewsbury. In contrast to Palo Alto, where divorce was rampant, there were very few divorced families in Shrewsbury. However, the boys' competence at school and participation in sports soon earned them respected positions in their peer groups. I also became accepted as the boys' mother and was recognized for my position at the Worcester Foundation, a respected local institution. However, I was careful that we did not stand out from the crowd. The Robinson grandparents were big fans of track and field. DanDad, as the boys called their paternal grandfather, had been an Olympic miler. He with MomMom (their paternal grandmother) attended all Olympics. When DanDad and MomMom invited Billy to join them for the 1980 Moscow Olympics, I felt he should not go. The US government had boycotted the Olympics because of the Russian invasion of Afghanistan. It was all right for the Robinson grandparents to go. They were well-known Olympic sports fans in their Indiana community. But it was not all right for us to go. In Shrewsbury, we were borderline outsiders and failing to boycott the Olympics would have made us real outsiders.

A central challenge for my life with the boys was meshing my family life with my scientific life. I had taken multiple months off after each birth, and as the boys grew, timed my working hours with their nursery school and then regular school hours. Now at the Worcester Foundation, my first full-time job since Billy's birth, I would work nine to five, being sure to be home for supper and the evenings. I also did not work weekends. But when I did work, I was totally focused on the work. The first summer that the boys went to visit their father, I was free to work more hours. I put in longer hours but rapidly discovered that I could not sustain the intensity that I put into work for more than eight hours and went back to eight-hour days with a swim in a local pond after work. My nonworking hours in the evening and on weekends refreshed my mind, allowing me to accomplish more than if I had been in the lab focused on the logistics of yet one more experiment. Putting the science part of my life into "idle" while I was with the boys let the science compartments of my brain consolidate and reassort.

Time flew as the boys graduated from Spring Street School and attended Shrewsbury Junior High School. When Billy, whom we now called Bill, was finishing junior high, Shrewsbury High

School held an open house for the parents of students who would be matriculating the following fall. Schooling in Shrewsbury had been more than adequate in elementary and junior high schools, and I was anticipating the same in high school. At the open house, I was taken aback by the announcement that the high school was going to have a four-day week with the goal that students receive practical work training on the fifth day. For the boys to have the benefits of a solid academic high school education, we would need to move to another school district or switch from public to private schools.

To identify a better high school for the boys, I went to the MIT admissions office to find out what schools near Worcester provided MIT with academically strong, well-trained students. They answered Westborough High, a public school, and Saint Mark's, a private boys' boarding school that took a limited number of day students. Following up on both leads, I began to hunt for a house in the Westborough school district and Bill applied for a day-student slot at Saint Mark's.

When Bill and I visited Saint Mark's, a golden retriever met us in the parking lot and proudly escorted us through the cloisters to the admissions office where we underwent separate interviews and tours. The school emphasized its sports as well as its academic programs. Teachers, virtually all male, included a mixture of recent college graduates as well as seasoned dons. It was a very male environment, ideal for boys being raised by a single mother. Bill was jubilant when he was accepted as a day student. Al and Tom were also accepted at the time they completed junior high. All three would become members of "the privileged, the proud and the few" as the day students called themselves. We were able to afford Saint Mark's because an educational trust in my family paid half of the cost. The remainder would be paid by me, the boy's father, and the boys (who made regular contributions to their tuition).

Once the three boys were going to Saint Mark's, I looked for and bought a house within walking distance of the school. The twelve-mile move from Shrewsbury to Southborough would be made after the boys were home from their summer activities, immediately before the fall term. Uncle Nick helped us move, which we did with fifteen loads in two pickup trucks. The last load included the woodpile. On arrival, Bull, our beloved dog, assessed the new yard and promptly marked his perimeters. The boys could now walk to Saint Mark's, which filled their lives with athletic as well as academic and social activities. We would no longer need Eunice, our live-in household help, who had been with us since our early days in Shrewsbury. The boys and I would take on Eunice's tasks.

We appreciated Saint Mark's. It provided so much more for teenage boys than could have been provided by a public school, Eunice, and me. Saint Mark's also appreciated us. Bill would become editor in chief of the school newspaper, Al would captain the lacrosse team, Tom would excel in academics as well as athletics and I would become head of the Parents' Association.

While we still lived in Shrewsbury, Wally had suffered a heart attack while driving out from Boston for our weekly Thursday dinner. Fortunately, he was near an emergency medical clinic where he pulled in and received immediate care. Despite the immediate care, his heart had been badly damaged, and he only partially recovered his pre-heart-attack vigor.

In the summer of 1986, before we moved to Southborough, Wally failed to appear at work and his concerned colleagues called his building manager who found him in his bed where he had passed in his sleep. The boys were at camp. Uncle Nick gathered the boys together after breakfast and told them of Wally's passing. Wally's brother, Mike, came up from New York and together we arranged for a service and the disposition of Wally's belongings. The furnishings that came to us, a leather couch, bookshelves, and books were the first furniture to be delivered to our new Southborough home. The day of the service, Uncle Nick and the boys drove down from New Hampshire.

The boys changed into their sports jackets and khaki pants in the funeral home parking lot; and, although Wally's brother invited us to sit in the family row, we sat just behind the family row. It was a Reform Jewish service; not short, but to the boys "so short, Mom." After the service I drove to camp, following the Camp Kabeyun van, so that I could have the solace of the boys for the weekend.

Later, Wally's brother Mike and I would take Wally's ashes to Vermont, where they were interred in the West Thetford Pleasant Ridge Cemetery. This cemetery contains the remains of my paternal grandfather, my great-aunt Azubah, who had helped with the education expenses for my father and asked that I be named Harriet, and most recently my father. It is where I have asked that my ashes be interred. The cemetery, on the crest of a hill next to a pasture with cows, is very peaceful. The graveside service would consist of Mike and me plus the gravedigger. We read psalms we had picked the night before, choking up as we read. The gravedigger asked us if we were all right. We soldiered on.

Wally had not belonged to a synagogue and there had been no one to help his brother and me with our grief, the service in

Boston, or the graveside service in Vermont. I did not want the boys to be in a similar position should something happen to me. I set out to join a church, first trying Southborough's Pilgrim Church, a Protestant church I could walk to. At the church, I not only found neighbors but a preacher who was delivering cogent messages. I began to join church activities. When a new preacher who gave dismal sermons became the pastor, I taught Sunday school so that I did not have to sit through the preaching. I had found a new group, a meaningful group, which helped fill the void left by Wally's death.

Wally's death left an enormous hole in our lives as we missed the weekly companionship that the boys and I had so enjoyed. Wally had been a central figure in my life for over twenty years. When he had broken up with me at the time I had received my master's degree at MIT, I had treated the emptiness by reentering the MIT graduate school to earn a PhD. By the time I was defending my thesis, Wally had reappeared. But I, with a new PhD, was headed west for postdoctoral training. At the collapse of my marriage, when the boys and I returned to Massachusetts, Wally again had reappeared. The boys could see that my parents and brothers knew and liked Wally and almost immediately accepted him, as if he were a special uncle.

Now Wally, in his death, had again had a major impact on my life, stimulating my return to an active church life. My family had been active in the church during my youth. I had then left the church during college, unsure of the dogmas. On my return, I did not take Communion. But after seeing the movie *Places in the Heart*, where the image of a deceased father sits in the pew with his family for Communion, I more fully joined the church by taking Communion. I value my church for the "love" it preaches, the music, and for taking me into a broader community than just scientists.

The boys' high school years flew by. Before we knew it, all three had graduated from Saint Mark's and been accepted at Stanford where they would graduate in the classes of 1989, 1990, and 1991. Going to Stanford meant they would be near their father, who purchased them a van, which they shared. Stanford did not send bills or grades to the parents, so I was minimally aware of their progress except for what they volunteered when home on vacations. All three had full and interesting college years. Bill and Tom were pre-med students while Al took engineering with a particular interest in the environment. Tom spent semesters abroad in West Berlin and Krakow (Poland) and worked one summer in South Africa where he travelled daily into the townships to help at a medical clinic. Bill started the Stanford Kayak Club, Al served as social director for the Whitman House dormitory.

Once Tom went to college, I had the world's worst case of empty nest syndrome, which was heightened by Bull, our beloved dog, contracting a hematological cancer and having to be put down. The hardest part was cooking for myself. I was a fast cook, but not cooking for the boys, I cooked less nutritious foods and began to slowly gain weight.

An invitation came from Stanford inviting parents to attend the fall parents' day. I bought a new suitcase, arranged to stay with Triebe, our neighbor from when we had lived in Palo Alto, and booked a ticket that would give me a weekend in Palo Alto followed by a week visiting Aunt Barbie in New Mexico. The trip was totally therapeutic. As soon as the boys appeared, I could tell they were happy. All three were wearing their flipflops. Tom's hair was down to his shoulders. I visited their rooms, and discovered that Oinks, a large stuffed pink pig (acquired from a thrift shop), had gone to college with Al. It was a fun weekend.

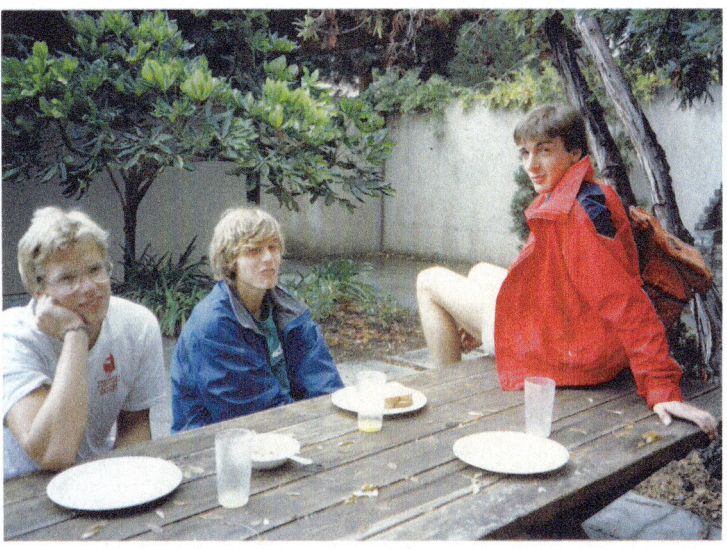

The Boys at Stanford's Fall Parents' Weekend —1987. From left to right: Al, Tom, Bill. We are in the backyard of Whitman House where both Al and his future wife Kathy lived. The boys drove a communal van that their father got them. All three, sitting in a row, took psychology together.

College expenses can be overwhelming. But paying for Stanford was less than paying for Saint Mark's because of the educational benefit (50 percent of tuition), that their father received as a Stanford Professor. My family's educational trust paid 50 percent of tuition plus 50 percent of room and board. According to the divorce agreement, their father paid two-thirds and I paid one-third of the remaining costs. The years of heavy educational costs for me had been the high school years.

After Stanford parents' weekend I proceeded on to visit Aunt Barbie. Aunt Barbie, now ninety-three, was living in a retirement community in Santa Fe. The community was within easy walking distance of the Santa Fe Plaza where native vendors displayed their jewelry and art. I visited the Plaza and bought the boys trinkets. Together, Barbie and I visited the Santa Fe gallery that sold her work, including paintings she had done while at her retirement community. I drove her to Taos where she and Uncle Howard had lived for more than fifty years to visit her former home with its view over an agricultural valley. We visited the Taos galleries displaying her work and the Taos Inn displaying Works Progress Administration murals painted by her and Uncle Howard. We ate at her favorite Taos restaurant.

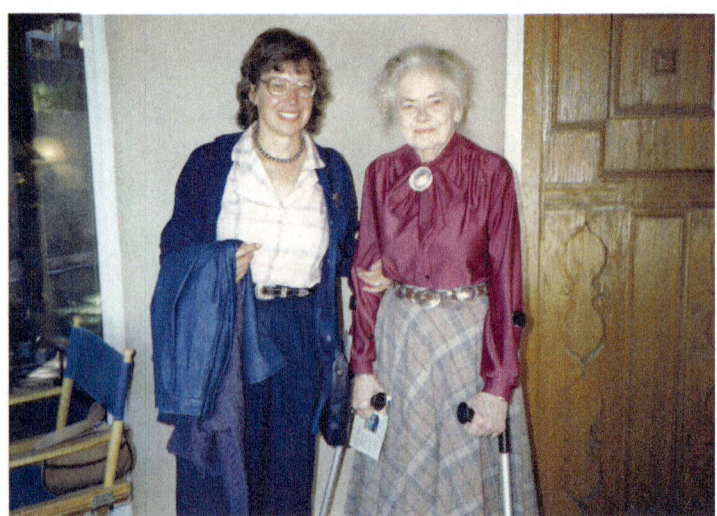

Visiting with Aunt Barbie, Barbara Latham Cook. She and Uncle Howard were part of the Taos art community. I am on the left and Barbie is on the right.

Just as the high school years had flown by, the Stanford years flew by. All three boys took a year off between undergraduate and graduate school. Bill worked in a Stanford lab. Al was a raft guide for the summer and a ski patroller at Deer Valley Utah for the winter. Tom worked at Genentech on the production line for tissue plasminogen activator and then wind-surfed in Hawaii. In Hawaii, he waited table at the Four Seasons.

Bill would go on to medical school at Stanford and as of early 2024 is Chief of Rheumatology and Immunology at Stanford. He is a founder or cofounder of companies developing antibodies as therapeutics. Al went to graduate school in Engineering at the University of California in Berkely and as of now is Dean of Engineering at Colorado State University. Prior to being a dean, he was an institute professor at Carnegie Mellon University where he was Chair of Mechanical Engineering and spent two years as Director of the Carnegie Mellon Campus in Rwanda. Tom would go onto medical school at Columbia University and is now Professor of Surgery and Vice Chair of the Aging Surgical Wellness Program at the University of Colorado School of Medicine. Prior to his current position he was Chief of Surgery at the Denver Veterans Administration Hospital. He is recognized for his contributions to geriatric surgery. They all have had the good fortune of both liking and thriving in their jobs. As the boys have grown, I also have enjoyed the good fortune of my jobs providing opportunities for advancement and the excitement of major waves of discovery. Meanwhile group adventure, marriage, and grandchildren have continued to enrich an ongoing family life.

PART II:
My Academic Years (1977–2008)

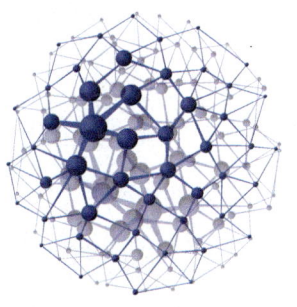

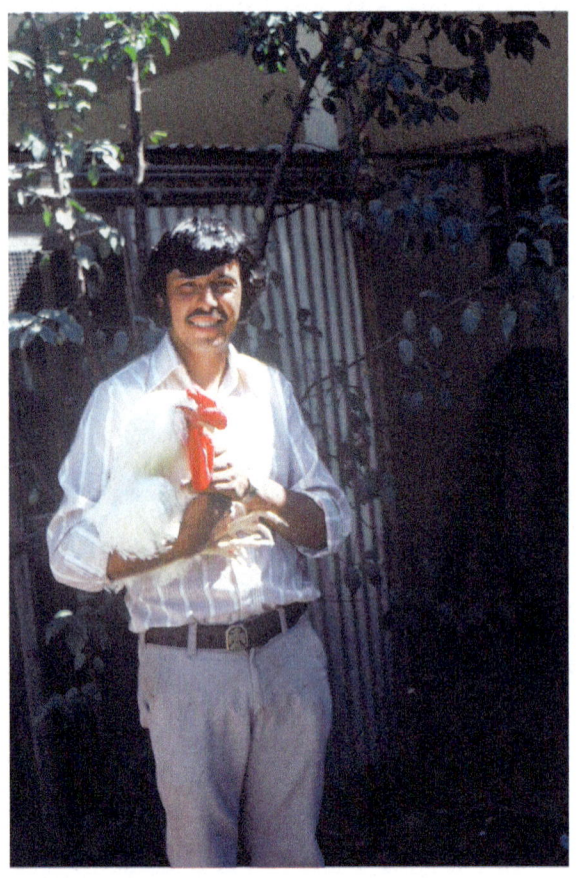

Rick Salazar Holding a Rooster. The Stanford Chicken shed is in the background. Rick was invaluable in helping me get my Worcester Foundation lab running and the chickens moved from California to Massachusetts.

CHAPTER 10:

Cancer Induction by Insertional Mutagenesis (1977–1987)

The Worcester Foundation for Experimental Biology would be the first place that I would have a lab of my own. Rick Salazar, who had originally worked in the research program at Kimber Farms and then moved to Stanford when Kimber Farms broke up, came to Massachusetts for two months to help me set up. He was invaluable, maintaining a clear focus while I was pulled in many directions. We found him a rental cottage within walking distance of the Foundation.

My first task in my new job at the Worcester Foundation was to move the chickens I had bred for chick-helper-factor from California to Massachusetts. I did this in the winter of 1977, as soon as the chicken facility at the Foundation had been completed. The different pedigrees were moved as embryonated eggs. Rick and I drove into Boston's Logan Airport to pick up the first shipment of eggs, only to have the dispatcher unable to locate our boxes. Dismayed, we said, "it's eggs," and the dispatcher instantly knew where he had placed them, in an area where they would be sure not to freeze. We were relieved, and even more relieved when the chicks hatched. The inseminations and packing of the shipment had been done by a research associate in my former husband's lab and the boys' favorite babysitter. The actual shipment occurred in a window of mild weather. The Worcester Foundation Public Relations Office let the *Worcester Telegram* know of the successful hatch. The newspaper sent their photographer, who took pictures of the chicks which were published on the front page. Something that nobody would have noticed at Stanford was newsworthy in Worcester, Massachusetts where the midwinter hatching of very cute chicks from eggs that had started in California caught the fancy of the townspeople.

Rick also helped with the second highest priority—getting the tissue culture going. Key to preparation of growth medium for cells is water quality. Millipore, a new biologics company, installed our water purification system. Following the lead of the installment engineers, Rick and I stood back when the newly plumbed system was turned on. The fittings held, no one got wet. Millipore also featured us, publishing a picture of us and our new water system in their company newsletter.

Rick's visit ended with a lab warming in the large empty space across the hall that with time would become my larger lab. We sent invitations with a sketch of a chicken serving hors d'oeuvres to the entire Foundation staff (about three hundred people) and set up my hi-fi system for background music. The Foundation still suffered a schism between those who had and those who had not supported the court case over salaries for women. Not everyone spoke to each other. But I was new, had kept my nose out of the schism, and had a new beginning to celebrate. Everyone came to what turned out to be a bash, the biggest party of my life. People throughout the Foundation learned who I was, welcomed me, and in the future would be ready to help me and my lab.

My initial studies at the Worcester Foundation built on my postdoctoral work and the chicken breeding I had done at Stanford while working part time when the boys were little. In my postdoctoral years I had shown that chicken cells infected with the Bryan strain of Rous sarcoma virus produced noninfectious virus-like particles. These particles became infectious if Rous sarcoma virus was grown in the presence of a Rous helper virus. In my Stanford years, I had shown that these particles also could become infectious if they were produced in uninfected chicken cells that were positive for chick-helper-factor. Could chick-helper-factor be genes for Rous helper viruses that had somehow gotten into chicken DNA?

In 1977, analyses for the presence of Rous helper virus sequences in chicken DNA were being pioneered by Susan Astrin at the Fox Chase Cancer Center outside of Philadelphia. In her work, Astrin had found that chicken DNA did indeed contain sequences related to Rous helper viruses. She detected these as bands of specific sized DNAs using a technique called Southern blots (see below). The question we were interested in was: Did the different patterns of chick-helper-factor that we had bred chickens for at Stanford correlate with different bands of Rous helper virus sequences in Southern blots of chicken DNA?

I invited Astrin to give a seminar at the Worcester Foundation. After her seminar, we set up a collaboration in which she would analyze the sizes of the bands of DNA related to Rous helper viruses in the chickens I had bred for specific patterns of chick-helper-factor. Immediate work would be on DNA extracted from frozen cells that I had typed for chick-helper-factor.

SOUTHERN BLOTS:

A Technique for Identifying Specific Sequences in DNA

In preparation for performing a Southern blot, DNA is purified and cut with restriction enzymes (functional proteins) that recognize and cleave specific 4 to 8 base pair sequences of DNA.

The cut pieces, which have many different sizes, are then fractionated for size using an electric current to sieve them through an approximately 10-inch long and 1/4-inch thick slab of agar (a form of gelatin). How far a DNA fragment moves reflects how long it is. Short pieces move further than long pieces. The sieved pieces are then transferred (blotted) from the agar to nitrocellulose paper, a type of paper that binds DNA.

Once on the paper, radioactive probes are used to identify the sizes of bands containing sequences of interest (in our case Rous helper viruses). The sizes of bands are determined by comparing how far a band had moved relative to marker bands of known size. The name Southern is for Jim Southern who first developed the technique.

The collaboration was highly productive. Almost immediately, we showed that specific patterns for the expression of chick-helper-factor correlated with specific bands of helper virus DNA in chicken DNA. These bands of helper virus DNA were termed endogenous viruses because they were being transmitted by chicken DNA. The term endogenous distinguished these viruses from exogenous viruses that are transmitted by infections. It turned out that chickens have lots of endogenous viruses related to Rous helper viruses (like ten to twenty) that are transmitted in the DNA of sperm and eggs. Only one of these endogenous viruses could produce infectious helper virus. All the rest had different partial sets of helper virus genes, a phenomenon that accounted for the different patterns of expression of chick-helper-factor.

The 1975 Nobel Prize shared by Howard Temin and David Baltimore would be awarded for studies that revealed the mechanism for the generation of endogenous viruses. These scientists showed that the RNA of Rous sarcoma virus (Temin) or the RNA of a murine leukemia virus (Baltimore) is copied into DNA as part of the normal life cycle of these viruses. The copying of RNA into DNA was termed reverse transcription to distinguish it from the heretofore held dogma that DNA is transcribed (copied) to RNA. RNA viruses that reverse transcribe their RNA to DNA as part of their life cycle were named retroviruses. In the retrovirus life cycle, the DNA formed by reverse transcription becomes inserted (integrated) into the chromosomal DNA of the cell that is undergoing infection. This inserted DNA is called a provirus. The endogenous viruses we were working with were Rous helper virus proviruses embedded in and being transmitted in germline (egg and sperm) chicken DNA!

Having identified the endogenous viruses in my chickens allowed me to breed all but one ubiquitous endogenous virus, out of my chickens. Breeding a line of chickens with only one endogenous virus would prove important to understanding how Rous helper viruses cause cancer.

Breeding For Endogenous Viral Loci

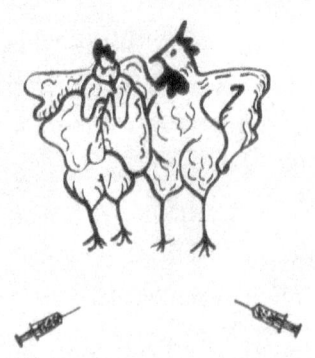

Erythrocyte DNA analysed for endogenous viral loci

Selective Breeding

Breeding Chickens for Only One Endogenous Virus. The breeding was done by artificial insemination, the pedigree of eggs marked and then clutches from the different matings hatched. In contrast to the cartoon, we, not the rooster and hen, chose who would mate with whom. Breeding for the absence of all but the near-universal chicken endogenous virus (ev-1), let us and others test for new proviral insertions associated with cancer.

In contrast to the Rous sarcoma virus that rapidly induces sarcomas in every single infected chicken, Rous helper viruses induce a variety of tumors (not just sarcomas) which occur in only a fraction of infected chickens and take months of sustained infection to appear. To study the mechanism for cancer induction by Rous helper viruses, I infected day-old chicks that I had bred to contain only one endogenous virus. Infecting chickens which had only one endogenous virus removed the background of endogenous virus bands to unmask new proviral insertions (caused by the infection) that might have played a role in cancer induction.

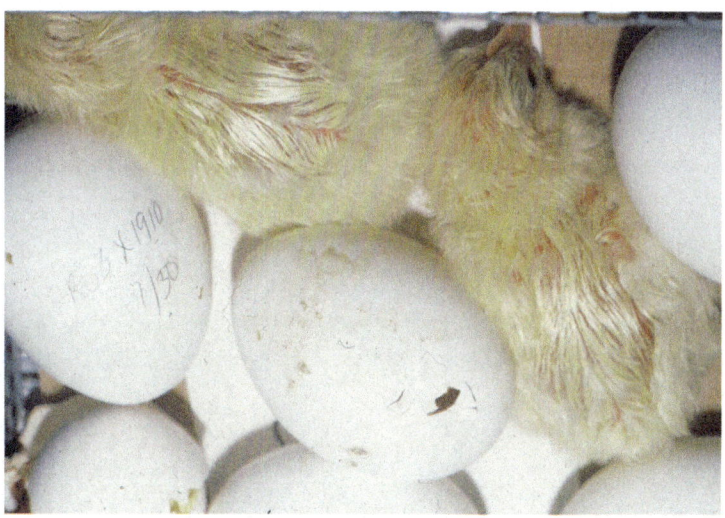

Hatching of Chicks for Cancer Studies. Day-old chicks, bred to have only the near-universal chicken endogenous virus (ev-1), were inoculated in the leg vein with Rous helper virus and then monitored for the appearance of tumors. The pencil markings on the eggs indicate the parents of the chicks. The chicks that have just hatched have not had time to fluff out yet. You can see the hole the chick immediately below the hatched chicks has pecked to begin its exit from its egg.

Bursal lymphoma is a relatively frequent cancer in chickens caused by Rous helper viruses. Bural lymphomas in chickens arise in the bursa of Fabricius, the organ in chickens where white blood cells mature into antibody-producing cells. It is an outgrowth of the large intestine located next to the cloaca. When the infected chicks reached three months old, we started monitoring their bursas for tumors using weekly rectal exams. When tumors appeared, birds were sacrificed and samples harvested for Southern blot analyses, virus isolation, and determination of the tumor type. At harvest, a "bird sheet" was filled out giving the wing band number (attached at hatching), the weight of the bird (determined using my baby scale), the weight of the bursal tumor (determined using a regular laboratory scale), the sites of metastases (most frequently the liver), and the freezer location of the saved samples. To gain expertise in tumor identification, I read the chapter on tumors in the textbook *Poultry Diseases* and

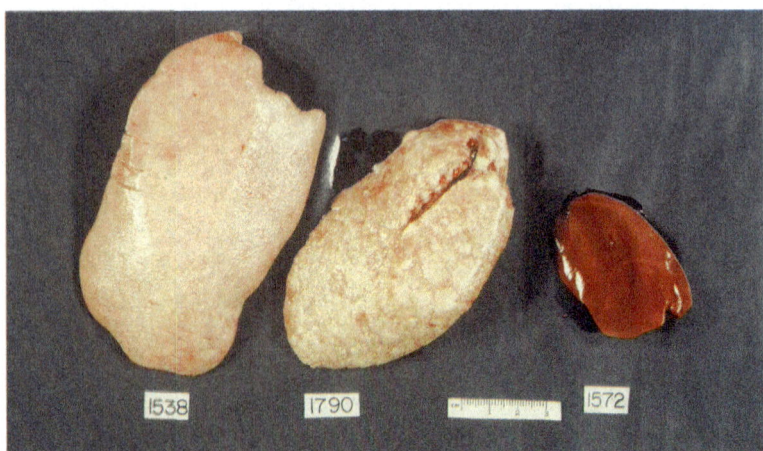

Examples of Metastases of Bursal Lymphomas. The lymphomas arose several months after inoculation with a helper virus. Metastases to the liver are shown for chickens 1538 and 1790. For comparison, a normal liver is shown for chicken 1572.

audited the hematology and pathology courses for medical students at the nearby University of Massachusetts Medical School.

The key analysis of the tumors, carried out by our collaborators as well as ourselves, would prove to be the Southern blot. These revealed proviral insertions (bands of helper virus sequences) next to the proto-oncogene *c-myc*. Proto-oncogenes are normal cell genes that are important for normal growth and development. However, if these genes are mutated for abnormal expression, they can become oncogenes, or genes that cause cancer. Analysis of the proviral insertions in the bursal lymphomas revealed insertions in the chicken proto-oncogene *c-myc*. These insertions had mutated *c-myc* to an oncogene. This new and exciting method of cancer induction was named "insertional mutagenesis."

More than one hundred cellular genes are now known to be able to be mutated by insertional mutagenesis, carcinogens, or radiation to become oncogenes. These proto-oncogenes code for proteins that affect cell growth and differentiation. At the time we started studies on retrovirus-induced cancers, the concept of cancer induction by the mutation of a proto-oncogene to an oncogene was new and not broadly accepted.

Cancer-inducing proviral insertions was an exciting and rewarding area of work that has proven to have relevance to human as well as chicken cancers. *C-myc* is deregulated in many types of human cancers with up to 70 percent of human cancers having deregulated *myc* expression. Where relevant, current cancer treatments test for and treat for the activation of specific proto-oncogenes to oncogenes.

My chickens had provided me with a unique and valuable niche for helping unravel how retroviruses cause cancer. My role in the demonstration that chick-helper-factor represented the expression of endogenous proviruses was seminal in the unveiling of endogenous viruses which are now known to exist in all species, including humans. Even more important, my collaborators and I helped to demonstrate that insertions of proviral DNA could cause cancer by mutating a proto-oncogene to an oncogene. Crucial to these studies were the Southern blots that enabled the identification of cancer-causing proviral insertions in chickens that I had bred to be largely free of multiple background bands of endogenous viruses.

As my work progressed and was published, I regularly attended, spoke at, and even organized the annual Cold Spring Harbor RNA Tumor Virus meeting. I was invited to join the editorial boards of the *Journal of Virology* and *Virology* and to be a section editor for *Virology*. I successfully supported the work of my lab with two major grants from the NIH—*Retrovirus-Host Interactions* and *Avian Leukosis Viruses and Cancer*—and became a member of and chaired national and state grant review committees.

I was rapidly promoted by the Worcester Foundation from staff to senior scientist and would become one of only a handful of principal scientists. With the promotions came higher salaries and a larger lab. I had also come to play a role in the greater Boston virology community where I spoke at, and helped organize, the Virology Dinner Club. This club meets once a month at Harvard for dinner followed by a seminar. Speakers from Harvard, MIT, Tufts, Brown, and the University of Massachusetts Medical School were picked based on the timeliness of their research.

By this time, I was lecturing in the virology course at the University of Massachusetts Medical School. I gave lectures to the medical students on retroviruses, hepatitis B virus, and herpesviruses. The coordinator for the medical school pathology course approached me to lecture to the second-year medical students on the role of retroviruses in cancer. I agreed and with the goal of the students appreciating that cancer was being caused by abnormal expression of normal cellular genes, had the students practice pronouncing the names of the growing number of newly identified proto-oncogenes: *c-src*, *c-myc*, *c-erb*, *c-myb*, and *c-fos*. This was sufficiently out of the ordinary that the students reported me to Dr. Majno, the Chair of Pathology, who called me into his office to find out what was going on. Rather than lambasting me, Dr. Majno was intrigued by my teaching new findings on the origins of cancer. At the end of the meeting, Dr. Majno initiated a recruitment process that would allow me to join his Department of Pathology as a research professor.

Dr. Majno's offer was very attractive. Not only would I be moving to a much more substantial institution than the Worcester Foundation, but I also would have access to the Biosafety level 3 containment facilities that were being built to allow study of a newly discovered retrovirus, HIV. The proximity of the Worcester Foundation and the medical school meant that I would not need to move the chickens, which could stay at the Worcester Foundation.

CHAPTER 11:
Pioneering Studies on DNA Vaccines (1989–1997)

My father had once told me that there had been two periods of creativity in his life. The first had been when he was a young engineer collaborating with his high school friend, Din Land, to make Polaroid's first product, polarized lenses for sunglasses. The second had been after his children had left home and he had focused on the development of blood processing equipment.

With the boys all now in college and my move to the University of Massachusetts Medical School complete, I also would enjoy a "late" highly productive and creative period in my career. At the University of Massachusetts, I would have two main labs, a dark room and space in a long connecting corridor for freezers. During the remodeling, I merged and pivoted the two main labs by ninety degrees so that the entrances to the labs would open onto a back corridor, which had windows. I then had a bank of desks built under the windows to give the staff a pleasant place to read and analyze data as well as have a reagent and virus-free space for eating and drinking.

The lab was ready in late January 1988. I scheduled the move for the second week in February. This move would involve a full staff and much more "stuff" than my move to the Worcester Foundation ten years earlier when Rick and I had arrived with three liquid nitrogen tanks with frozen cells and a large dry ice shipping box with frozen stocks of virus packed in gallon paint cans. This time, lab equipment, glassware, and notebooks would be packed by fellows, staff, and students as well as professional packers.

It was snowing on the day of the move, just as it had been ten years earlier on my move to the Worcester Foundation and fifty years earlier on the day of my birth. The Foundation was close enough to the medical school to allow the freezers to be unplugged, moved, and immediately plugged back in with little risk of the contents thawing. At the end of the day, surrounded by unpacked boxes, the lab staged a surprise birthday party for me. They brought out a cake and lit up the candles. To the group's horror, a still smoldering match disappeared into a ventilation intake. Luckily, nothing caught fire. Dave Brown, a senior fellow, then produced a present, a subscription to *Wrestling* magazine to be delivered to me at the medical school. Fortunately, it was a joke, and I would not have pictures of near-naked brawny men regularly arriving in my departmental cubby.

Once at the medical school, my areas of research expanded to include work on vaccine development, which grew out of my work with Rous sarcoma virus in chickens. Work with Rous sarcoma virus had shown that viruses could carry and express nonviral genes, such as *c-src*. My initial vaccine work would replace the *src* gene in Rous sarcoma virus with the influenza virus hemagglutinin gene, which encodes the viral spike protein that is the main target for protective antibody.

In our first trial we explored whether Rous sarcoma virus in which the *src* gene had been replaced with the H7 avian influenza gene could protect against challenge (exposure) to a lethal H7 avian influenza virus. To test whether our recombinant H7-expressing virus could protect chickens against an H7 influenza virus challenge, I contacted Rob Webster at Saint Jude's Children's Hospital in Memphis, Tennessee. Webster oversaw a high-level containment facility (Biosafety level 4) where he could conduct lethal H7 influenza virus challenges without risking the infection spreading to and causing disease in wild birds or commercial chickens. All the vaccinated chickens—but none of the unvaccinated—survived exposure to the lethal H7 virus. The H7 expressing retrovirus had expressed sufficient H7 protein in inoculated chickens to serve as a protective vaccine for H7 influenza virus.

Our first test had been with a replication-competent form of the H7 expressing virus that could spread in an inoculated chicken. We next tested whether a replication-defective form of the H7 expressing virus could provide protection. A replication-defective virus would be a safer vaccine because it could infect a chicken but not spread in the vaccinated chicken or be transmitted to another chicken. Successful vaccination would depend on the original infected cells expressing sufficient H7 protein to be able to stimulate protective immunity. The replication-defective virus achieved protection, showing that a replication-defective virus could express sufficient H7 protein to provide protection!

In both trials, recombinant DNA had been used to make the H7-expressing viruses. Infectious viruses produced by the recombinant DNA had then been used for vaccinations. Recovery of infectious viruses was done by introducing (transfecting) the recombinant DNAs into cultured cells. Once in the cell, the DNA could express RNA that in turn would code for the proteins that formed the virus. The transfected cultures produced the viruses that Webster used for vaccination.

The next step was to test whether the recombinant DNA, itself, could be used to vaccinate without going through the step of recovering infectious virus in cell culture. Introducing DNAs into cultured cells had been facilitated by chemicals that would be too toxic for use in whole animals. Therefore, we used as much DNA as we could make for inoculations.

Larry Hunt, a sabbatical fellow, prepared three different DNAs for testing: DNA for the replication-competent Rous virus expressing influenza H7 in the place of *src*, DNA for the replication-defective Rous virus expressing influenza H7 in the place of *src*, and DNA for the Rous virus without a *src* or H7 DNA insert (the control). Because we did not know what route of inoculation might be best, Webster inoculated test chickens by three different routes: intradermal (into the skin), intraperitoneal (into the abdominal cavity), and intravenous (into a vein). Webster doubted that sufficient DNA would be taken up in a whole chicken to produce protective levels of the H7 protein. But given that our earlier vaccines had worked, he went ahead and inoculated chickens with the candidate DNA vaccines. I knew the vaccination had worked when a stunned Webster left the phone message: "Send more vaccine."

Webster's message was left on September 9, 1991. By September 11, I had filed a patent disclosure with the University of Massachusetts Medical School, called "Immunization by Inoculation of DNA Expression Vectors into Animals." We had our notebooks notarized and set to work making more DNA. Webster ordered more chickens. In the second trial, only the DNAs coding for the replication-defective virus and the control DNA were tested as vaccines. The second trial confirmed the first trial and again showed that the DNA producing the replication-defective H7-expressing virus elicited protection. We did not tell a soul what we were doing until a patent had been filed on March 23, 1992. Once we had the patent filed, we could talk about our findings, only to find that no one believed us.

Despite the excitement of discovery, 1992 was a hard year. My first choice for publishing our results was *Nature*, the prestigious British weekly. The *Nature* editors were intrigued but their reviewers considered the results "fireworks." How could sufficient DNA have been expressed in a whole animal to elicit a protective immune response? Immunizations with proteins used milligrams of protein. Inoculated DNA expressed mere micrograms of protein—a thousand times less than required when inoculating proteins. Based on two sets of negative reviews, the editors had to reject the manuscript, but they were curious and invited me to speak at the December 1993 *Nature* conference in Amsterdam, "From DNA to Drugs." For my presentation. I wore my bright red suit so that those interested in talking to me could easily spot me after my presentation.

I resubmitted our manuscript, this time to *Science*, a prestigious American weekly. The *Science* reviewers, too, did not believe the results were possible and rejected the manuscript.

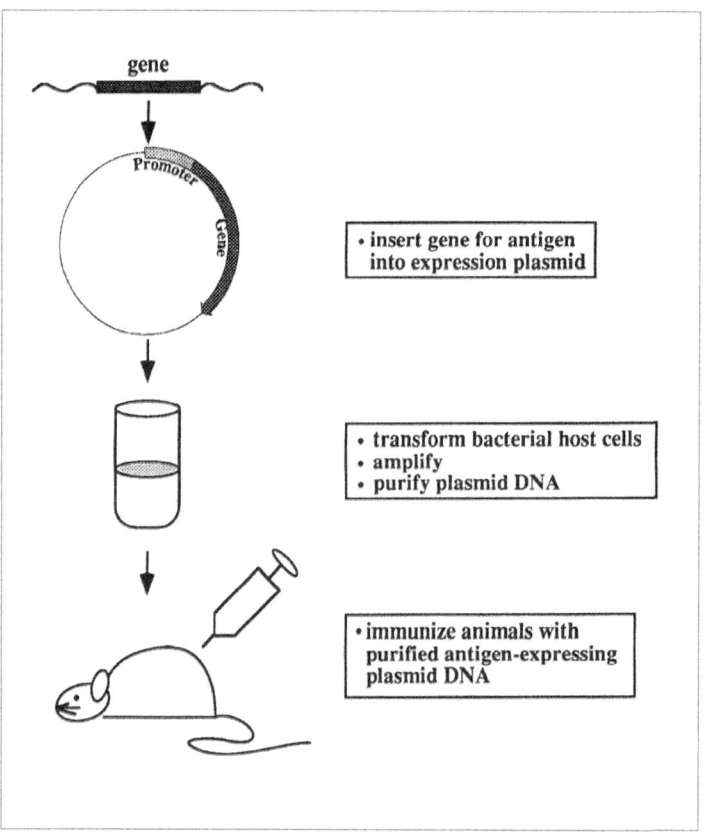

Schematic Depicting the Development, Production, and Inoculation of a DNA Vaccine. The gene (depicted in black) is the DNA sequence for the protein one wants to use as a vaccine. The gene is introduced into an expression plasmid using recombinant DNA technology to create the vaccine. Plasmids are circular molecules that self-amplify in bacteria. An expression plasmid is a plasmid that has been engineered to contain an appropriate promoter (depicted in grey) for expression of the introduced gene in cells. The expression plasmid containing the vaccine gene is introduced (transformed) into bacterial cells and the transformed bacteria grown to amplify the vaccine plasmid. The vaccine plasmid is then purified from the bacteria, dissolved in a salt solution (saline), and directly inoculated into an animal to vaccinate the animal.

My next submission was to *Vaccine*, a specialty journal. The reviewers for *Vaccine* accepted the results but requested more detail on how Webster had done the injections, an easy revision. The revised manuscript was accepted October 10, 1992, but was not issued as a publication until August of 1993. I have never forgiven *Vaccine* for this timeline. I was not the only player in the new field of DNA vaccines and dates of publication are important gauges for the timing of discovery, although not as important as dates for filings of disclosures and patents, where my filings were the earliest for protective DNA immunizations.

But even harder than getting manuscripts accepted was obtaining competitive research funding. The competing renewal for my major NIH research grant was turned down in the spring of 1992. Later, the study section which had triaged the grant held a special session to educate themselves on DNA vaccines, and the Nobel Prize winner who had led the assault on my grant, entitled "A New Method of Vaccination," apologized to me for not having recognized the value of what I was doing. When all was said and done, the lab and I wrote nine grant applications to get two. The first successful grant was from the US Department of Agriculture, which was willing to gamble on the possibility of our work opening a new approach for the much-needed control of influenza infections in chickens.

Desperate for funds, I went to Dr. Majno, my department chair, and showed him our DNA vaccine data. He recognized the potential (as opposed to the impossibility) of what we were doing, and after consulting with the senior research faculty in the department awarded us $100,000 in departmental funds to keep us going. To conserve funds, I discontinued the chicken work. At my last chicken talk, in early December 1992, I choked up. My chickens had been my lifeline. My lab had worked with the chickens and the Rous helper viruses at a time when my results helped pioneer the genetic basis of cancer. I had made a difference. I had cared about my work with the chickens. There is still at least one lab using the chicken model to identify new oncogenes. But I moved on to work on the basic mechanisms of DNA vaccines and the practical development of a vaccine for HIV.

Despite the very modest interim funding supplied by the department, the lab—reduced to a single technician, Joe Santoro, and two fellows: Ellen Fynan, supported by an NIH fellowship; and Shan Lu, supported by a Howard Hughes Fellowship—was exceptionally productive. We were opening a new field, and like being the first into a blueberry patch, there was much to be picked. The creativity at the lab spilled over to having babies, with Joe, Ellen, and Shan all adding a firstborn to their families. In the future, I would show their pictures with

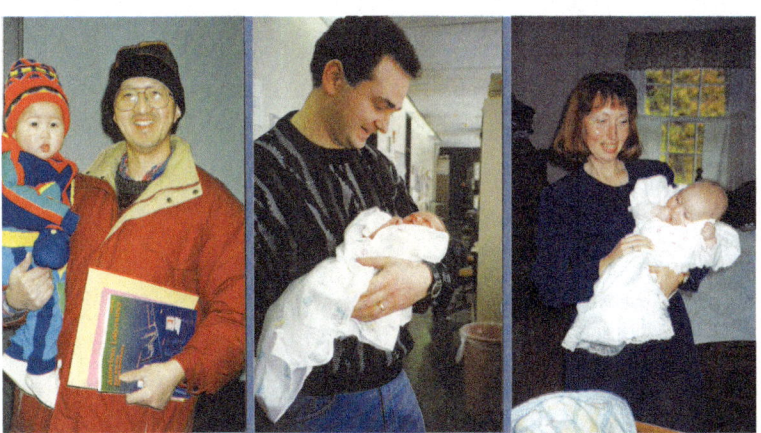

Lab Babies. From left to right: Shan Lu with his son Roger, Joe Santoro with his daughter Adrianna, and Ellen Fynan with her daughter Francis.

their babies in the acknowledgments section of my talks to let young aspiring scientists know that active careers are not incompatible with having a family.

Meanwhile, I submitted an abstract for our DNA vaccine data to the Eleventh Annual Meeting of the American Society of Virology to be held in the summer of 1992 at Cornell University. Webster was one of the organizers for this meeting. To maximize my audience, he placed my talk immediately after a "state-of-the-art" address that was anticipated to draw a full house. After I presented my data, the first question was an opinion: "You don't think this ever will be useful, do you?" I was discouraged, but did not give up, as what we were doing was simply too exciting to give up.

When I returned to the lab, I submitted an abstract for the September 1992 meeting, Modern Approaches to New Vaccines, including Prevention of AIDS, to be held at the Cold Spring Harbor Laboratory. This laboratory, on Long Island, was led by Jim Watson, who as a fellow had worked out the structure of DNA with Francis Crick. It is a mecca for molecular biologist. In my abstract, I used initials for my first name to avoid advertising that I was a woman. Prior to my session, when I gathered at the podium with the other speakers, the scientific organizer said, "so you are the author of this abstract, we were wondering who had done this work."

By this time, there was a small cadre of us developing direct DNA inoculations for vaccination. Stephen Johnston was the first into the field when his lab discovered that the growth hormone DNA he was testing for gene therapy, instead of making mice grow faster, was raising antibody responses. Vical Inc., a San Diego biotech firm, had licensed the use of direct DNA inoculations to express proteins in animals based on findings of Jon Wolf at the University of Wisconsin. Wolf had found that "naked" DNA (purified DNA with no additives) could produce proteins after direct inoculation into muscle. Phil Felgner at Vical was testing the ability of various liposomes (drug delivery systems) to enhance DNA uptake and expression in muscle. Merck Inc. in an effort led by Margaret Liu, had licensed the use of intramuscular injections of naked DNA for vaccination from Vical. David Weiner at the University of Pennsylvania was using an additive (bupivacaine) to enhance vaccination by intramuscular inoculations of DNA. The audience crowded around our handful of DNA posters. We talked until we were hoarse. We compared notes with each other on the DNA constructs and inoculation formulations we had tried, establishing the beginnings of relationships, some of which would become long-term friendships. The logjam for the acceptance of DNA vaccines had begun to break.

Three meetings were particularly important to the new field of DNA vaccines. The name for the "new" technology was chosen at a meeting convened by the World Health Organization in Geneva in the spring of 1994. At this meeting the technology was named "DNA vaccines" as opposed to "gene vaccines" (my favored name) or "polynucleotides in a vial" (Merck's favored name). A second important meeting was sponsored by the FDA. At this meeting, the safety of DNA vaccines was addressed, and the stage set for the FDA issuing *Points to Consider* guidelines for the manufacture and use of DNA vaccines. The third meeting, held in Atlanta in April of 1993, was the annual meeting of the American Society of Microbiology. What was notable about this meeting was not just the packed auditorium, but the audience's opinions and questions extending through the lunch break. Our DNA vaccine session would have gone even longer had the audience not entered the room for the post-lunch session.

NAMING OF NEW TECHNOLOGY, WORLD HEALTH ORGANIZATION, MAY-18, 1994

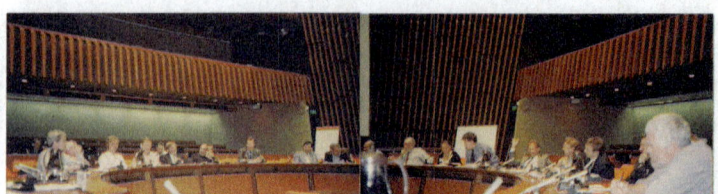

NUCELIC ACID VACCINES: DNA VACCINES, RNA VACCINES
Choice of a name that reflected the technology not modifying the germ line

Naming of the New Technology, May 18, 1994. Meeting at the World Health Organization where the new approach to vaccination was named DNA vaccines. I took the picture from the head table where I was seated. You can see my microphone!

It was exciting to see how easily this new technology could be used. All one had to do was make a vaccine DNA (a recombinant DNA) using one's own or commercially available expression vectors (DNAs designed to express inserted genes), introduce the DNA into an appropriate bacterium for the production (growth) of the recombinant vaccine DNA, purify the vaccine DNA and inoculate the desired host. Any protein for which one had a DNA sequence, any designer protein that one had conceived as being potentially useful, could be readily tested for vaccination in animal models.

When I attended the annual meeting of the American Society of Virology at Cornell in the summer of 1992, I had conserved our limited laboratory funds (the lab was being financed by the department at that time) by staying with a college friend, a professor in the Department of Botany. Chatting over breakfast, she told me about a gun that was being used to shoot DNA into plant cells. New traits were being introduced into plants, which have thick cell walls, by loading DNA expression vectors for plant proteins onto minuscule gold beads and then shooting them into cultures of plant cells. I was intrigued and went to visit the scientist who was shooting DNA into plant cells only to find that he was working in his raspberry patch. Later, I reached him by phone. He told me about a company, Agracetus, Inc., that was developing a gun for shooting DNA into mammalian cells. I contacted Agracetus, which called their technology "Accell particle bombardment." The company was very interested in our trying their technology and assigned Joel Haynes and Deborah Fuller to help us.

By this time, I had moved our studies into mice, which we were immunizing with an H1 hemagglutinin gene and using an H1 influenza virus for challenge infections. I had shifted to mice because of the ease of using large numbers of animals, the many reagents for studying immune responses of mice, and the ability to use an H1 influenza virus challenge under Biosafety level 2, rather than the high containment Biosafety Level 4 required for work with H7 influenza viruses in chickens. Our experiments used BALB/c mice, a sociable and curious strain of white mice, which if you are not watchful, pop out of their cages, just like popcorn.

Agracetus shipped me an Accel device, a machine the size of a refrigerator, with a gun port about the diameter of a quarter in the middle of a twelve-by-twelve-inch flat surface. My lab followed the Agracetus protocols to load DNA onto gold beads and then layer the beads onto mylar discs which fit into the gun port. The abdomen of an anesthetized mouse was shaved and treated with Nair, a depilatory agent. The mouse was placed over the port, abdomen down. My staff put on ear protectors and fired the electric discharge of the gun. The mouse lifted off as a boom reverberated throughout the Department of Pathology. To my relief, the procedure did not seem to bother the mouse. Five minutes later it was awake and exhibiting its usual curiosity. After this first inoculation, my lab held mice over the gun port by hand so that mice would not lift off with the gene gun shots.

My first experiment with the gene gun was to vaccinate mice using beads carrying different doses of DNA. The outcome of this experiment was that I could raise antibody with 250 times less gene gun-delivered DNA than I needed to use when delivering DNA using a needle and syringe. The gene gun proved to be a valuable experimental tool. However, despite the ability to use small amounts of DNA, particle bombardment has not advanced for medical use. Loading the gold beads with DNA is tricky and the DNA comes off the beads if exposed to even low levels of humidity. The gun, itself, has been substantially simplified and is now handheld and run using blasts of compressed helium instead of electrical discharges.

The development of the mouse model allowed me to ask a series of basic questions about the ability of DNA-based immunizations to raise humoral (antibody-mediated) cytotoxic T cells (white blood cells that can recognize and kill cells infected with a virus) and helper T cells (white blood cells that provide growth factors for antibody-producing cells and cytotoxic T cells). My lab was able to test the effects of gene gun versus intramuscular saline injections on the elicitation

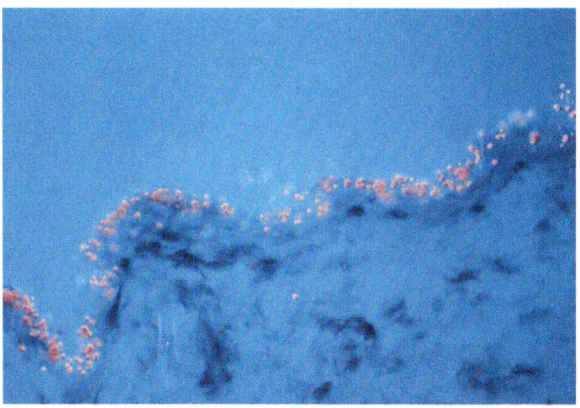

Section from a Gene Gun Inoculation Site in Mice. The small pink beads are the gold beads used to deliver DNA. The dark cells that vary in shape include immune system cells responding to the immunization. It is the take up and expression of the expressed vaccine protein by the immune system cells that raises the vaccine response.

of antibody and cytotoxic T cell responses and to examine the durability of elicited responses. I tested different forms of DNA-expressed proteins for the ability to elicit responses: secreted proteins, proteins displayed on the outer membranes of cells, and intracellular proteins. And finally, I explored the ability of DNA vaccines to prime and boost conventional vaccines, such as live-attenuated vaccines, inactivated vaccines, viral-vectored vaccines and protein-based vaccines.

Funding was no longer an issue as I readily obtained grants. The lab refilled with students and post docs. Dr. Majno was pleased with the results of his emergency funding and the University of Massachusetts featured me in its public relations. Ellen and Shan went on to positions as assistant professors. Joe moved to a senior technical position at Merck. My lab and I had had a year of exciting science that had placed us at the forefront of early-stage vaccine development.

CHAPTER 12:

Research Toward an AIDS Vaccine Using Rabbit and Macaque Models (1989–2008)

In 1990, when I was pioneering the use of DNA for vaccination at the University of Massachusetts Medical School, a new, inexorably fatal disease had appeared in homosexual men. This disease, which came to be known as acquired immunodeficiency disease (AIDS), was caused by a previously unknown retrovirus, HIV.

I had begun studies on this newly discovered virus using the Biosafety Level 3 containment facilities at the University of Massachusetts Medical School (U. Mass.) before my actual move to U. Mass. My goal in these initial studies was to identify an HIV envelope protein (Env) that could elicit antibody that would neutralize (block) HIV infections. For these studies, I worked with Eva Maria Fenyo of the Karolinska Institute in Sweden. Eva Maria had collected serial isolations of HIV from infected patients. These isolates contained samples from the multiyear pre-disease phase of infection as well as from the short, terminal AIDS phase of infection. Eva Maria had found that viruses from the pre-disease phase of infection had slow/low growth characteristics, whereas viruses from the terminal phase of infection had rapid/high growth characteristics.

To test how Envs with different growth characteristics affected the ability to elicit neutralizing antibody, my lab constructed DNAs expressing secreted monomers (termed gp120s), secreted oligomers (termed gp140s) as well as membrane-bound forms of Env (termed gp160s) from serial HIV isolates from patients number five and six. My lab also made candidate DNA vaccines for three isolates of HIV that

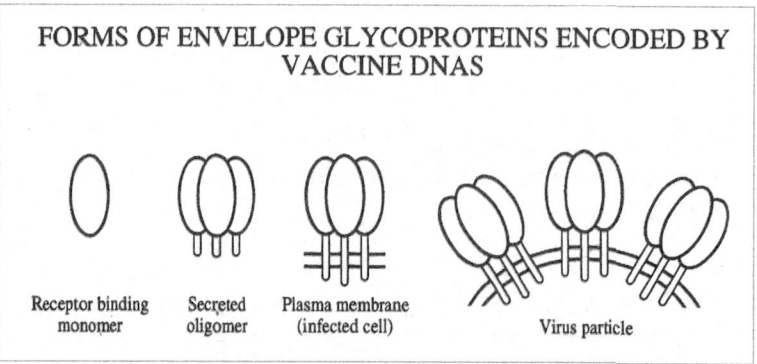

Schematics of Different forms of Env Tested for the Ability to Elicit Neutralizing Antibody. From left to right the schematics show a gp120 monomer (the globular receptor binding subunit of Env), a secreted gp140 oligomer (the globular receptor binding subunit plus a truncated form of the transmembrane subunit of Env), and the gp160 form of Env (the globular subunit plus complete transmembrane protein of Env displayed on the surface of infected cells and mature virus). The 120, 140, and 160 size designations are for one out of the three monomers that make up an Env spike. Gp stands for glycoprotein. The mature Env protein is heavily coated with sugars (glycosylated). This glycosylation provides camouflage from the immune system.

had been adapted for growth in cultured cells. In all I had thirty different DNA constructs for the study. To test for the ability to elicit neutralizing antibody, I used the gene gun for immunizations because such required so little DNA. My lab inoculated rabbits instead of mice so that we could obtain adequate blood for in-depth analyses of antibody responses.

Env proved to be poor at raising neutralizing antibody. The growth characteristics of patient isolates did not affect the ability of Env proteins to elicit antibody. Serial isolates of Env from patient five, irrespective of their growth characteristics, raised anti-Env antibody whereas serial isolates from patient six, irrespective of their growth characteristics, failed to elicit much anti-Env antibody.

However, the form of Env did affect the ability to elicit neutralizing antibody. Among the tested forms, the membrane-bound gp160 form of Env displayed on infected cells and virus-like particles raised the best (albeit low) levels of neutralizing antibody. The laboratory-adapted isolates raised antibody, but this antibody had poor neutralizing activity for patient isolates. Based on these data, we used patient Envs expressed in their natural gp160 form, displayed on the plasma membranes of cells and noninfectious virus-like particles for further vaccinations. My lab had identified a modestly favorable form of Env for raising neutralizing antibody but had not identified an Env that could raise broadly neutralizing antibody for patient isolates. Identifying such an Env remains the central unsolved challenge for those still working on vaccines for AIDS.

For me to work meaningfully on the development of an HIV vaccine, I needed to test the candidate vaccines I was making in an animal model where we could assess the ability to prevent AIDS by a challenge infection. A major constraint in AIDS research is the limitation of the ability to study actual infections to monkeys and apes. The most frequently used model is the study of simian immunodeficiency virus (SIV) infections in monkeys.

In October 1992, the NIH AIDS Task Force invited me to speak to them about the new field of DNA vaccines. At the suggestion of Frank Ennis, a professor in the Division of Infectious Diseases at U. Mass, who had served on NIH task forces, I prepared a one-page memo proposing a SIV DNA vaccine trial in macaques. During the lunch break, I handed my memo to Alan Schultz, who was overseeing NIH-sponsored nonhuman primate studies. As I was leaving for the airport, Alan caught up with me to let me know that there were nine monkeys that had been left over from an adjuvant (immune enhancer) study that could be made available for my use. Not only were they available, but they were located at a contractor in Worcester. I was elated.

My first SIV DNA vaccine trial (1992–1994) would compare gene-gun-only inoculations with three simultaneous routes of inoculation: gene gun, intramuscular and intravenous, for the ability to raise immune responses and protect against an intravenous challenge with SIV. The SIV DNA vaccine (a five DNA vaccine) elicited both anti-SIV antibody and anti-SIV white blood cells. At six weeks after the administration of the viral challenge, blood cells of both vaccinated groups showed five-times lower levels of SIV infected cells than the unvaccinated placebo group. But by twelve weeks post challenge, this protection had been lost and the levels of SIV infection were similar in the vaccinated and placebo groups.

I received the twelve-week post challenge data on Long Island where I was about to speak on DNA vaccines at Stony Brook University. I added the disappointing data to my presentation. Both Alan Schultz (our NIH Program Officer) and I had been impressed by the antibody and T cell responses the SIV DNA vaccine had elicited. But these had not protected the macaques. In this first trial, I had chosen a challenge virus (SIV251) that is fatal to macaques within months as opposed to the multiyear time course that is seen in typical human AIDS. I had chosen this challenge to be able to compare the control elicited by DNA with that elicited by live-attenuated vaccines. Live-attenuated vaccines can protect against SIV-induced AIDS. However, these are too dangerous for real-world vaccines because of the ability of the live vaccine to acquire mutations that increase virulence (allow them to cause AIDS) . In our next trial, we would lower the bar for potential success by using a more benign challenge infection.

Our second vaccine study in monkeys (1996–1999) used newly developed chimeras of SIV and HIV for both immunization and challenge. These chimeras, called SHIVs, allowed me to test vaccines expressing HIV (not SIV) Envs for immunizations and the relatively benign SHIV-IIIb virus for challenge. This trial had eight groups of four monkeys to test intradermal and gene gun inoculations of SHIV DNAs both with and without boosting with SHIV DNA, SHIV fowl pox vectors or a purified HIV Env protein. The DNA vaccine consisted of five DNAs and the poxvirus boost of three recombinant fowl pox viruses. A single SHIV-IIIb Env was used for the protein boost. Eight immunizations were given over sixty-six weeks. Challenge with SHIV-IIIb was at peak vaccine response, two weeks after the final immunization.

This second trial, which had used everything in our arsenal and had set a low bar for the challenge, revealed intradermal saline injections of DNA followed by recombinant poxvirus boosters providing protection. Post challenge, seven of the twelve monkeys primed with intradermal inoculations of DNA had no evidence of infection. In contrast, 11 of 12 animals primed by gene gun inoculations were infected. The best protection, three out of four animals, was in the group primed by intradermal DNA inoculation and boosted with the recombinant fowl pox vectors.

To test the durability of the protection, protected animals were rechallenged with SHIV-IIIb at forty-three weeks after their first challenge. The protection held. Nineteen weeks later, protected animals were challenged again, only this time with a SHIV with a different HIV Env, SHIV-89.6P. Four out of six of the intradermally primed animals remained uninfected.

Before leaving the second trial, I tested whether I could detect occult infections in the "protected" animals. To test for occult infection, blood was collected from the four protected animals and 10 ml (about two teaspoons) intravenously inoculated into naive monkeys. Two of the protected animals did not transmit an infection while the third transmitted the final SHIV-89.6P challenge and the fourth transmitted the earlier SHIV-IIIb challenge. These results clearly showed that my vaccine had not prevented occult infections, although it was certainly holding such infections at low levels.

In the second trial, I had rolled the dice for success by using matched sequences in the immunogens and challenge virus, and a relatively benign virus for the first two challenge infections. The fruits for this approach had been a clear indication that of the eight tested regimens, saline injections of DNA followed by a recombinant poxvirus boost, had the highest potential for protection. The study was accepted for publication in the prestigious journal, *Nature Medicine*, where it was featured on their fifth anniversary cover. I had achieved durable control of infection that did not depend on the presence of neutralizing antibody, a type of antibody that has been virtually impossible to raise for the HIV pandemic. The results of the second trial meant that I would go forward in further macaque trials using saline injections of DNA for priming and recombinant poxviruses for boosting. I would also begin preparations of HIV (not SHIV) vaccines for human trials that would use saline injections of HIV DNA for priming and recombinant HIV poxviruses for boosting.

In the winter of 1997, out of the blue, I received a phone call from Tom Insel, the new Director of the Yerkes National Primate Research Center at Emory University in Atlanta Georgia. Insel had recently joined the primate center and was recruiting faculty. He had called seeking my recommendations for faculty candidates with expertise in DNA vaccines. Without hesitation, I said that I, myself, would be interested in a position at the primate center. My first two monkey studies had been done at contract facilities where one does not have one's hands on the levers. If I was to effectively move forward with the monkey model for HIV vaccines, I needed more direct and flexible access to nonhuman primates.

Insel had not thought of me as the candidate; I was turning sixty. But he did invite me to give a joint talk to the staff of Yerkes and the nascent Emory Vaccine Center. During my visit, I was impressed with the favorable living conditions for the nonhuman primates, which being in Atlanta, a moderate climate, were largely outdoors. Being part of a vaccine center would also give me greater exposure to expertise in immunology than I had at U. Mass. Over the next few months, I heard nothing from Insel.

Meanwhile, Aventis Pasteur had licensed my DNA technology from the University of Massachusetts Medical School. I also had become a regular speaker at the annual Cent Gardes conferences sponsored by the Mérieux Foundation in Paris. Out of these contacts came a $400,000 award for work with DNA for an HIV vaccine.

During this time, I was regularly attending church and enjoying Sunday dinner with my father and his eighty-six-year-old bride whom he had married after my mother's death. During Sunday dinner I brought up the award and my limitations in using it at U. Mass. "Grandad," ever practical and always relevant, asked, "What would you really like to do?"

I answered, "use it for monkey studies at Yerkes."

He said, "write to them and let them know of the award and your interest in using it at Yerkes."

The next day I sent a brief handwritten note to Insel. Unbeknownst to me, the candidate who had been the first choice for the job had just turned down Insel's offer. My note reopened my candidacy.

As the recruitment became serious, I realized that I was afraid of the South. Even in Atlanta, a progressive southern hub where citizens are "too busy to hate," Northerners, easily recognized by their accents and even dress, were considered aggressors by the local population. Despite my fears, I accepted the offer to be Chief of Microbiology and Immunology at the Yerkes Primate Research Center, with my first year to be a sabbatical year so that I could meet the ten-year requirement to vest my State of Massachusetts pension.

The primate center was in turmoil as Insel transformed it from a stodgy backwater housing nonhuman primates to a modern research institute. As part of team-building, Insel hired a social psychologist to conduct a series of retreats. My first contacts with Yerkes, outside of recruitment, would be attending these off-site weekend sessions. Harold McClure, who flew American flags out of both front side windows of his car with the script, "these colors don't run," had been the previous Chief of Microbiology and Immunology. Insel had created a new division, Comparative Pathology, that McClure would lead when his original position was transferred to me. Screwing up my courage, I sat next to McClure at the first and subsequent retreats. As I began to get to know McClure, I found that I was sitting next to a man who was not only totally dedicated to his work, but a gentleman who pushed in my chair at lunch and opened the doors for me. During the retreats, McClure and I became a team.

As I moved back and forth between U. Mass. and Yerkes during my sabbatical year, McClure was an enabler. Working together, we increased the size of my first monkey study at Yerkes by keeping the macaques at the Yerkes field station during the vaccination phase of the trial. The field station had a much lower per diem (daily fee) than the main station, where the challenge infections would be conducted. I came to respect McClure and the care he afforded the monkeys, and he appreciated me because he recognized that I was seriously interested in my use of the Yerkes macaque resource.

During my sabbatical year, my lab remained at U. Mass. pending the completion of the new Vaccine Research Center building that would be attached to the Yerkes main station. My Division of Microbiology and Immunology would occupy the top floor of the new center. While the construction was ongoing and my pension was vesting, I alternated two weeks in Massachusetts with two weeks in Atlanta. While in Atlanta, I rented a room from a Delta flight attendant who bought and flipped houses on the side.

During my time in Atlanta, I began to get to know the Microbiology and Immunology staff I had inherited. Using my start-up funds, I purchased an overhead projector to project data from transparencies. Such were widely used for group meetings before the advent of PowerPoint. Group meetings are venues for presentation and discussion of ongoing research. The first

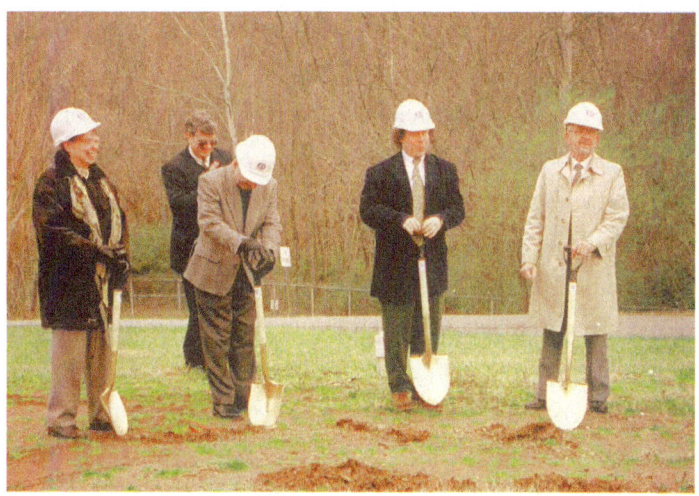

Breaking Ground in January 1998 for the Emory Vaccine Research Center. From left to right: me, Rafi Ahmed (Director of the Emory Vaccine Center), Mark Feinberg (Current Director of the International AIDS Vaccine Initiative), and Harold McClure (Director of Comparative Pathology). I still have my shovel, mounted on my bedroom wall.

group meeting was treated by the presenter as an opportunity to have bagels. I gave the second meeting to provide a model for presenting and discussing ongoing research. I also started division seminars, inviting the faculty of the Vaccine Center as well as faculty from the adjacent US Centers for Disease Control (CDC) to speak. From these informal seminars I learned who was doing what.

The actual move of my lab from Massachusetts took place before the new vaccine center building opened. This move was into temporary space on the first floor of the primate center next to the director's office. My office was on the third floor with the veterinarians and neuroscientists. This was cumbersome, but I did get to know the veterinarians and Insel (the director) came to know my lab, which was running full steam.

My third macaque trial (1998-2001) would build on our second trial at U. Mass. where saline injections of DNA followed by poxvirus boosters had durably controlled a series of challenge infections. For the third trial, my lab constructed a new SHIV vaccine using SHIV-89.6 sequences. This new vaccine used only one DNA, not the five DNAs used in previous studies. I wanted to develop a practical vaccine, one that would be easy to manufacture.

Since a poxvirus boost would be used for our DNA prime, I called Bernie Moss, a colleague from graduate school days, for advice on which poxvirus vector to use. Bernie, an expert on the use of poxviruses to express genes to be used for vaccination, recommended that we use modified vaccinia Ankara (MVA). The parent poxvirus for MVA was a smallpox vaccine that had been attenuated by donkey-calf-donkey passage at the Ankara Vaccination Station in Turkey. In the 1950s, the Germans undertook further attenuation of the Ankara vaccine, a vaccine which saved lives but had side effects, by subjecting it to 570 sequential passages in chicken cells. During its passage in chicken cells the Ankara vaccine lost its ability to replicate in mammalian cells where it undergoes an abortive infection in which it expresses poxviral proteins but does not produce progeny virus. This attenuated smallpox vaccine became MVA, a smallpox vaccine with minimal side effects that could be safely used in immunocompromised humans.

In our second trial at U. Mass., I had used three fowl poxvirus vaccines for our poxvirus boost. Linda Wyatt, an associate of Bernie, would make us a single, multiprotein-expressing MVA vaccine. Both our DNA and Linda's MVA vaccines displayed the HIV 89.6 Env on virus-like particles. This was the form of Env my lab had found to be most (albeit only modestly) effective at eliciting neutralizing antibody in rabbits.

Given a DNA prime-poxvirus boost vaccine had achieved durable vaccine-mediated protection in the second trial at U. Mass., the first trial at Emory would test a challenge at seven months post-vaccination, not the previously used two weeks. At two weeks post-vaccination, vaccine responses are at peak levels. By seven months they have contracted into memory, mimicking the conditions a vaccine would need to face in the real world. Also, to make the challenge a closer mimic of natural infections, which occur mainly through sexual activity, I had the veterinarians use intrarectal challenges, not the intravenous challenges used in the two earlier trials in monkeys.

I held my breath as samples came in post-challenge. Would infection be prevented? If infection was not prevented, would it be controlled? Infection was not prevented. But the memory responses of the vaccinated animals sprang into action, controlling the infection to background levels. The soaring immune responses preserved CD4 helper cells and the architecture of the lymph nodes, both of which were destroyed in the unvaccinated animals. The nonvaccinated monkeys progressed to AIDS while the vaccinated monkeys remained healthy. The manuscript reporting the third study (the first conducted at Emory) was published in April 2001 in *Science*, where it briefly became a most cited study in immunology.

I had gone from working with chickens to working with nonhuman primates. Chickens have personalities, but these personalities are not nearly as close to human personalities as monkey personalities. One of the rules at Yerkes was that the caretakers did not give the monkeys names. Despite this, the veterinarians became attached to their charges, and did give names. The most memorable of these was ValuJet, named after a low-cost airline that crashed due to improper stowage of flammable materials. ValuJet was an adolescent male who was always scraping himself as he moved from cage to cage through his social tunnel. Great emphasis was placed on housing friends with friends and ensuring appropriate medication and timely euthanasia for those developing AIDS. The NIH and the Emory Institutional Animal Use and Care Committee reviewed all trials. The moral responsibility of the researchers was to only conduct trials where the results had true hope to improve control of human disease. I worked with nonhuman primates not because I liked working with monkeys, but because it was the only challenge model for human AIDS vaccines.

On the next page I summarize the important findings of my three major macaque trials that determined the immunogens and regimen I would take forward in humans.

\multicolumn{4}{c}{The SIV Vaccine Trials in Macaques that Determined the HIV Regimens to be Tested in Humans}			
TRIAL	TEST VACCINE	CHALLENGE INFECTION	FINDING
1st U. Mass. 1992-1994	SIV DNA-only (9 macaques)	SIV251 intravenous challenge at two weeks after the last boost	DNA alone did not protect
2nd, U.Mass., 1996-1999	SHIV-IIIb DNA priming followed by DNA, fowl pox, or protein boosting (32 macaques)	SHIV-IIIb intravenous challenge at two weeks after the last boost followed by late SHIV-IIIb and SHIV-89.6P challenges	DNA followed by a poxvirus boost was more effective than DNA alone or DNA plus a protein boost, Priming with saline injections of DNA was more protective than priming with gene gun inoculations
3rd Yerkes (Emory) 1998-2001	SHIV-89.6 DNA priming and MVA boosting, MVA priming and boosting (36 macaques)	SHIV-89.6P intrarectal challenge at seven months after the last boost	Failed to prevent infection but both DNA-MVA and MVA-MVA vaccines showed excellent long-term control of the challenge infection by memory responses

There was a tremendous amount of satisfaction in conducting the SIV vaccine trials. Working with my lab and Bernie Moss and his lab, I had not only simplified our immunogens from five DNAs to one DNA and from three poxvirus vectors to one poxvirus vector, but I had also determined that I should use saline (not gene gun) inoculations of DNA and poxvirus (not protein) boosts. I would now prepare for human trials. This would require making HIV immunogens modeled on my SHIV immunogens. It would also require working under good laboratory practice (GLP) and good manufacturing practice (GMP) conditions that are required for pharmaceuticals destined for inoculation into humans.

In the third and last part of this autobiography, I recount the formation of GeoVax, Inc., a company focused on taking my DNA-MVA virus-like-particle vaccine into human trials. GeoVax was founded in 2001. I would work one day a week at GeoVax until 2008 (Emory faculty are allowed to devote 20 percent of their effort to consulting). In 2008, at the age of seventy, I would become emerita at Emory and a full-time employee of GeoVax.

PART III:
My Entrepreneurial Years (2001-2019)

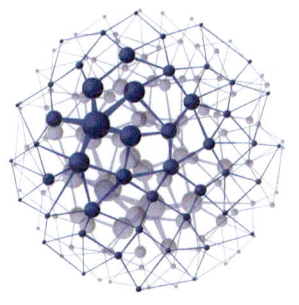

CHAPTER 13:

Cofounding and Serving as Chief Scientific Officer of GeoVax (2001–2017)

From the very early days of DNA vaccines, as far back as 1992, I had wanted to start a company to help move DNA vaccines from the bench to the bedside. Such was not possible at the University of Massachusetts where state employees were prohibited from licensing technology that belonged to the state (my patents for DNA vaccines, which had been developed at U. Mass., belonged to Massachusetts). A similar restriction was not held at Emory, a private university. The newly formed Emory Vaccine Center was supported in part by the Georgia Research Alliance that had been championed by Governor Zell Miller to attract biotech to Georgia by fostering academic "Centers of Research Excellence". The Emory Vaccine Center was one of these Centers. The Georgia Research Alliance had helped recruit Rafi Ahmed to lead the Vaccine Center through provision of an Eminent Scholar Endowed Chair and had helped get the new Vaccine Center off the ground by purchasing state-of-the-art equipment for the Center. Flow cytometers for enumerating white blood cells and DNA sequencers, luxuries that one didn't even dream of using outside of closely controlled central facilities at U. Mass., were available for individual use at Emory. The Research Alliance had even planned an incubator laboratory for start-up companies and was well positioned to support my interest in founding a company.

Ahmed, the Director of the Emory Vaccine Center, arranged for me to go before the leadership team of the Emory Woodruff Health Science Center and the Emory Medical School to present my HIV vaccine research and my interest in forming a company to commercialize the vaccine. The outcome of the meeting was that the Health Science Center and the Medical School would provide $750,000 to help get the company off the ground.

I now needed a Chief Economic Officer (CEO) who would supply business acumen for the company. A lawyer whom I had worked with on filings for the Emory DNA patents suggested Don Hildebrand who had led the development of veterinary vaccines at Rhone Mérieux Inc. in Athens, Georgia. Hildebrand lived in Athens, the home of the University of Georgia, about seventy miles east of Atlanta. Hildebrand was now retired, but active as a consultant. Hildebrand came to Atlanta to review my data. It turned out that he had overseen manufacture of experimental DNA and poxvirus-vectored veterinary vaccines. He was intrigued and signed on for the job. He would live in Atlanta during the week, returning to Athens on Thursday afternoon for a long weekend.

Hildebrand and I named the company GeoVax for Georgia vaccines. Geo was chosen because it had the entendre of "worldwide" as well as being the first three letters of "Georgia." The company logo was chosen to imply a globe, and when sufficient space was available, included the slogan: "Vaccines Serving Humanity." In 2002, exclusive rights to the designs of the DNA and MVA vaccines that my collaborators and I were developing were licensed to GeoVax in an interinstitutional agreement between Emory, the NIH, the CDC, and GeoVax.

The initial charge for GeoVax was to oversee the funding, licensing, manufacture, and regulatory issues needed to take our candidate DNA-MVA HIV vaccines into clinical trials. These vaccines would be modeled on the single DNA, single MVA SHIV vaccines that had showed such promise in my third nonhuman primate trial (see Chapter 12). Both the DNA and the MVA vaccines would express noninfectious virus-like particles displaying the natural gp160 form of Env that I had found raised the best, albeit weak, neutralizing antibody for HIV.

Because GeoVax was developing vaccines for human clinical trials, both the DNA and MVA vaccines needed to be developed and produced under GLP and GMP conditions. GLP and GMP practices minimize the potential for chance contaminants being engineered into a vaccine or becoming hitchhikers in vaccine preparations. GLP work is done by trained workers in a dedicated space, with defined reagents following rigorous protocols documented by detailed worksheets and regular review. Not all researchers, especially academic researchers, have the patience or rigor to work under GLP conditions. The initial staff Hildebrand brought into the company had worked in industry under GLP conditions and readily transferred this rigor to GeoVax, setting the standards that would be used to train further staff. As soon as the GeoVax Lab was operative, work on the DNA constructs was moved from Emory to GeoVax so that it could be conducted under GLP conditions. While at Emory, it had been conducted under "GLP-like" conditions using dedicated work benches with dedicated reagents according to defined protocols.

GLP work at the Moss lab, which is located at the NIH in Bethesda, was conducted in a locked room with dedicated reagents and a parental strain of MVA that had been sequestered and frozen in 1974 before the appearance of bovine spongiform encephalopathy (mad cow disease). Because the fetal calf serum used in the growth medium for MVA is at risk for harboring bovine spongiform encephalopathy, all passages of this 1974 MVA and its derivatives had been and are still being conducted using irradiated sera from Australia and New Zealand, two countries that are free of bovine spongiform encephalopathy.

GeoVax's initial home would be in the incubator lab that the Georgia Research Alliance had helped fund. Located on the Emory Briarcliff campus, a campus that had originally been an estate and then a mental hospital, the incubator consisted of seven trailers connected by a roofed walkway. An administrator occupied the first trailer that provided a front desk, a waiting room, and a lunch space. The remaining trailers were set up as laboratories, with the second trailer housing common equipment. GeoVax initially occupied the third trailer, but as the company grew, expanded into the fourth and fifth trailers. Payroll and benefits were handled by an outside contractor.

The very first staff included Hildebrand and three of his former employees: Jack Berg, who oversaw laboratory work and the development of manufacturing protocols; Mark Keister, who handled contracting and regulatory submissions; and

Michael Hellerstein, who did analytic assay development and validation. I spent one day a week at GeoVax, consistent with my employment agreement at Emory. At GeoVax, I managed and applied for government grants, helped with patent preparation, and worked with Hildebrand on fundraising.

The staff at GeoVax developed analytical methods to be used for product release and stability testing. Some of these tests were validated (tested for reproducibility) at GeoVax while others were transferred to appropriately audited contract facilities for validation testing and use. Reference standards for comparison of manufactured products with the original product were created for both the DNA and MVA vaccines. GMP storage facilities were vetted and a facility for storage of the vaccines chosen.

Manufacture of the DNA and MVA vaccines used contract facilities built to meet guidelines for GMP manufacture. These facilities, which are regularly audited by the FDA and the European Medicines Agency, were audited by GeoVax immediately prior to our use. Methods for manufacture were piloted at the GeoVax Lab and then transferred to the GMP labs for trial runs. For actual manufacturing runs, a GeoVax observer would be in place at the GMP facility. At the time GeoVax needed GMP manufacture for Phase 1 and Phase 2 trials, the United States had a dearth of facilities qualified for small-scale GMP manufacture of biologics. We ended up using facilities in the former East Germany and Scotland for our initial GMP DNA and MVA products, respectively.

During its first five years, GeoVax would successfully oversee the contract manufacture and testing of the DNA and MVA vaccines for first-in-human trials of our DNA vaccine and of our DNA prime followed by an MVA boost vaccine.

As the company moved its candidate DNA and MVA vaccines into clinical trials, my role evolved into serving as the GeoVax liaison with the clinicians and staff who were conducting the trials. I also worked hard on building collaborations for clinical testing of the vaccines we would make for Africa and India.

In January 2006, to increase the ability to raise funds, Hildebrand took GeoVax public through a reverse merger with Dauphin Technology Inc., a publicly traded company with defunct business operations. The merged companies would be called GeoVax Labs, Inc. After the merger, the shareholders of GeoVax and Dauphin would hold 67 percent and 33 percent respectively of GeoVax Lab's outstanding stock. Emory University would become the largest shareholder of GeoVax stock, owning about 31 percent. The Board of GeoVax Labs, Inc. would initially have two directors designated by Dauphin's

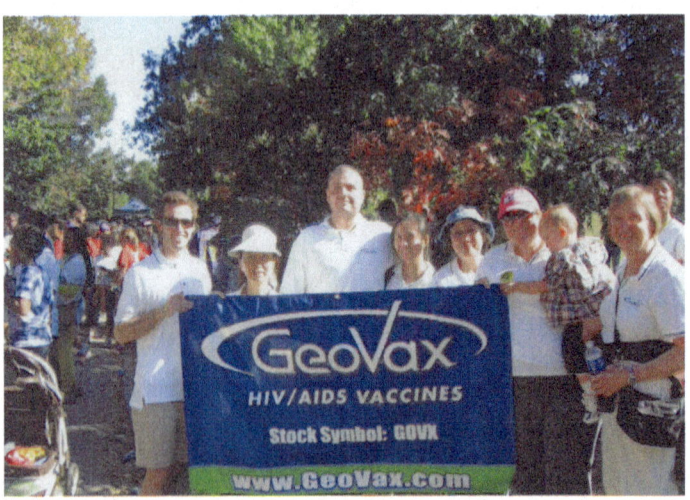

GeoVax Staff and Families Marching in the Annual Atlanta Gay Rights Parade. We are wearing our GeoVax polo shirts. I am at the far right. Note our stock symbol on the banner.

management and four by GeoVax. At the closing, Dauphin was to supply $13 million in cash as operating capital for GeoVax Labs Inc.

Although going public was done to facilitate raising funds, the reverse merger had downsides, the most damaging of which was Dauphin providing only a fraction of the cash, about $3 million of the $13 million, that was supposed to have come to GeoVax on closing. The former CEO of Dauphin also proved to be very hot-tempered and disruptive. He constantly pushed for the issuance of unrealistic press releases on the progress of the GeoVax vaccine, undoubtedly to support his efforts to raise the funds which Dauphin was supposed to have secured prior to the merger.

Going public also had the disadvantage of requiring detailed quarterly disclosures of financial activity and progress on company milestones. For a small company like GeoVax, it would have been preferable to have remained private until we were more advanced in product development and closer to having a product we could sell.

GeoVax would have three different CEOs during my time with the company. The first, Don Hildebrand, a cofounder, was CEO from 2001 to 2008. The second, Robert McNally, was CEO from 2008 to 2018; and the third, David Dodd, from 2018 to present. Both McNally and Dodd had been members of the board before becoming CEO. Each of the CEOs brought a different style to running the company. Hildebrand placed his emphasis on manufacture of the needed products for clinical trials. He was extremely frugal but an enormous amount of fun to work with. When he handed the reins to McNally, the reins came with a bank account of several million dollars. McNally was a manager. He oversaw the move of the company from the incubator facility to biotech space on Atlanta's ring highway. He cleaned up the board by accepting the resignation letters of the disruptive Dauphin members (which they used as threats and had not intended to be accepted). He moved annual meetings to the "Board Room" in the corporate offices of our legal counsel. Our patent lawyer was changed from a Boston firm to an Atlanta firm. During most of McNally's tenure, the company continued to focus solely on HIV vaccines, which were falling out of favor with investors because of the failures of early efficacy trials testing Genentech's gp120 protein vaccine and Merck's viral vectored vaccine. At the time Dodd took over, the executives and board were working for reduced (or no) pay, and what limited private funds were coming into the company came through the sale of convertible preferred stock in amounts insufficient to sustain the company. On taking over, Dodd focused on cleaning

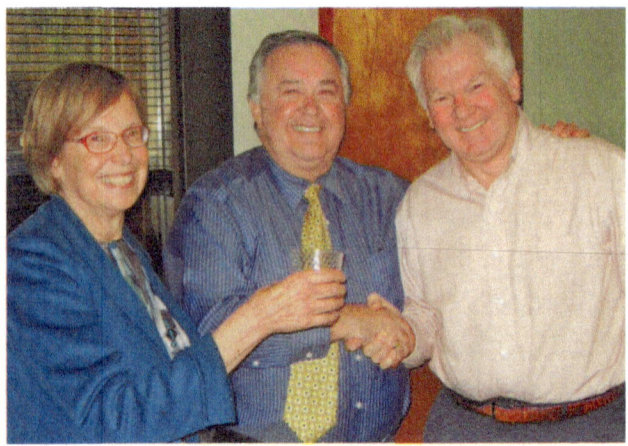

Senior Staff of GeoVax. Left to right: Me with Don Hildebrand and David Dodd. Don was a cofounder with me and the first CEO. David is the third CEO.

up the capital structure of the company and raising funds, which was helped by the company's entry into the COVID-19 vaccine space. These efforts culminated in a $12.8 million public offering and NASDAQ listing of the company's common stock in September 2020, with over $50 million subsequently being raised during 2021 and 2022.

Throughout the early years of the company I served in several roles, most importantly as a member of the board of directors and as Chief Scientific Officer (CSO). As my eightieth birthday approached, I became CSO emeritus to free the CSO position for my successor. For continuity for the company, I would visit GeoVax monthly and remain on the board of directors for a year after my retirement.

CHAPTER 14:

Development of GeoVax DNA and MVA HIV Vaccines (1998–2006)

The initial development of the GeoVax DNA and MVA vaccines was a collaboration between Emory, the NIH, and the CDC. In this early development, we had used chimeras of human and simian immunodeficiency virus (SHIV) sequences for vaccine constructs so that I could assess the ability to raise protective immunity using live virus (SHIV) challenges in macaques. I also had evaluated DNA constructs expressing different Envs and different forms of Env in rabbits to determine the form of Env that had the best ability to elicit neutralizing (blocking) antibody for HIV. These early studies had led to advancing candidate DNA and MVA vaccines that expressed noninfectious virus-like particles displaying the natural form of Env on their surfaces. These noninfectious particles raised antiviral antibody and cytotoxic (killer) T cells against the two major proteins of immunodeficiency viruses: Env and Gag. Elicited antibody against Env had the potential to block incoming infections, whereas elicited T cells against both Env and Gag had the potential to kill cells that had become infected by virus that had made it past the antibody.

The AIDS pandemic was initiated by a virus in chimpanzees undergoing chance infection and spread in humans. As HIV spread from its initial transmission, it evolved into clades (subtypes) defined by geographic clusters of distinct sequences. In 2001, GeoVax set out to construct and establish the collaborations for testing vaccines that would cover three of the major infections in the world. These included a circulating recombinant form of clades A and G (termed AG), clade B, and clade C. AG is a West African virus where HIV is speculated to have originated by exposure of people to infected blood during the preparation and consumption of bush meat. The CDC had collected DNA sequences for the AG virus and was particularly interested in working with GeoVax on making an AG vaccine. Clade B is the dominant infection in the United States, Europe, Australia, and Japan, where it has spread by sexual contact, particularly homosexual contact, and intravenous drug use. Clade C, the dominant clade worldwide, is present in sub-Saharan Africa and India where it has spread primarily by heterosexual contact and intravenous drug use. DNA sequences for a clade B and a clade C vaccine were available in an AIDS repository at the NIH.

GeoVax modeled its AG, B and C HIV vaccines on the SHIV vaccines that had controlled the SHIV challenge infection in my third trial in nonhuman primates, a trial conducted at Yerkes (see Chapter 12). These SHIV vaccines had used a single DNA and a single MVA to express noninfectious virus-like particles. Because GeoVax was making vaccines for humans, Jim Smith, a fellow, introduced additional safety mutations into the candidate DNA vaccines to ensure that the expressed virus-like particles could not become an infectious virus. These mutations also ensured that chance recombination of the GeoVax DNA vaccine with a circulating virus would inactivate the circulating HIV. In all, ten mutations ensured that exposure to the HIV DNA vaccines could not cause an HIV infection.

In addition to being safe, it was important that the GeoVax vaccines express high levels of virus-like particles (the immunizing proteins) and be suitable for large scale manufacture. These attributes varied for different AG, B and C sequences. In all, seven clade B sequences from Europe and the United States, four recombinant AG sequences from West Africa, and four clade C sequences from sub-Saharan Africa and India were screened to identify the B, AG, and C DNAs to be advanced in candidate DNA vaccines. During the selection process, each candidate DNA vaccine was introduced into mammalian cells to test for the level of expression of virus-like particles. Each candidate DNA was also serially introduced into bacteria to screen for stable high-level growth of the vaccine DNA.

Once the candidate DNA vaccines had been constructed, the DNA sequences were sent to Linda Wyatt in the Moss laboratory at the NIH for construction of matched AG, B, and C MVA vaccines. The candidate MVA vaccines were tested in both the Moss laboratory and at GeoVax for high levels of production of virus-like particles. Both labs also subjected the MVA vaccines to serial passage in chicken cells to test for the stability of the vaccines with passage. The clade B and clade C MVA vaccines constructed by Wyatt produced high levels of virus-like particles and were stable with passage. The AG MVA candidate, however, was not stable, losing its gp160 Env sequences with passage. This vaccine was reengineered to express the secreted oligomeric gp140 form of the AG Env, a form that was stable with passage. DNA and MVA vaccines that had completed vetting were moved, as funding allowed, into seed bank production, analytic testing, and trial runs for GMP manufacture.

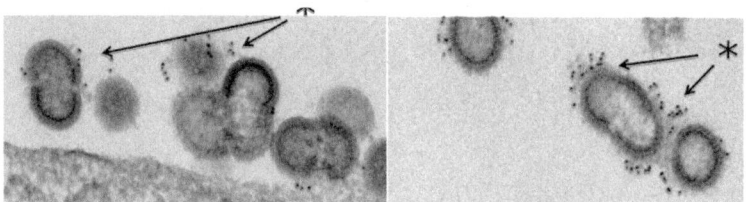

VLPs expressed by DNA prime   VLPs expressed by MVA boost

* Immuno-gold staining for native Env

Electron Micrographs of the Virus-Like Particles (VLPs) Expressed by the GeoVax Clade B DNA and MVA Vaccines. Cells expressing the vaccines were harvested, fixed, and stained with gold beads that had been charged with antibody that recognized (would bind to) the Env protein. The cells were then thinly sectioned for electron microscopy. The small gold beads in the micrographs indicate the presence of Env on the surfaces of the VLPs.

CHAPTER 15:

Clinical Trials of GeoVax's HIV Vaccines (2001–2019)

In parallel with the construction and preparations for manufacture of the AG, B, and C HIV vaccines, I worked on building the collaborations that GeoVax would need for testing the vaccines in humans. For the clade B vaccine, the collaboration would be with the US NIH-sponsored HIV Vaccine Trials Network (HVTN). For the AG recombinant virus, I would work with the CDC and the First Lady and Ministry of Health of the Ivory Coast in West Africa. For the clade C vaccine, I would work with the Indian Department of Biotechnology under the umbrella of a US-India Vaccine Action Program. All three efforts started in the early 2000s, but moved toward fruition at different speeds, much like the race between the hare and the tortoise in Aesop's fables. Below, I recount our work toward testing two "hares": the AG and C vaccines, which jumped out of the gate but did not make it into human trials, and one "tortoise": the clade B vaccine, which plodded out of the gate, but *did* make it into human testing.

Testing the AG Vaccine in the Ivory Coast (2001–2002)

In 1988, the CDC and the Ivoirian Ministry of Health formed a collaboration for work on HIV called Project Retrovirus Côte d'Ivoire (Projet RETRO-CI). By 2001, Projet RETRO-CI had more than one hundred employees and was conducting clinical trials on the ability of antiretrovirals administered at the time of birth to prevent mother-to-child transmission of HIV. As part of their clinical program, Projet RETRO-CI had determined the prevalence of HIV in women visiting antenatal clinics in the ten regional capitals of the Ivory Coast. These frequencies ranged from a high of 12 percent to a low of 7.7 percent, discouraging frequencies for the Ministry of Health, but highly favorable frequencies for obtaining end points in clinical trials.

Given the urgency of its epidemic, in April of 2001, the Ivory Coast convened a six-day meeting on HIV vaccine development. Because of my work with the CDC, I was invited to attend and speak. In preparation for the trip, the CDC Travel Department vaccinated me for yellow fever and equipped me with their standard West African medical kit: mosquito repellant, a prophylactic anti-malarial to be taken daily, rehydration salts for diarrhea, and antibiotics. We flew into the capital, Abidjan, known as the "little Paris" of Africa, on Air France, the airlines of their former colonial master. Under the first president of the Ivory Coast, who had held office for thirty-three years, the country had prospered in an otherwise turbulent West Africa. As I was driven from the airport to the Hotel Ivoire, I passed through a city not unlike midsized cities in the United States. The hotel, a twenty-four-floor high-rise, was a bit worn, but modern and with amenities such as restaurants, pools, and a gym. It was next to a state-of-the-art convention center where the workshop would take place.

On my first day in the Ivory Coast, there was an orientation visit to Projet RETRO-CI, which was located on the campus of the main hospital for Abidjan. This clinic included examination rooms for testing, counseling, and treating people with AIDS, clinical and basic science laboratories, and a data management center. Particularly impressive among the staff was John Nkengasong, Chief of the virology section, who was leading studies on maternal-to-child transmission. The orientation day was followed by a two-day International Workshop on HIV Vaccine Development and then a final two days for an in-depth review of Projet RETRO-CI by the CDC participants and sightseeing by the GeoVax participants.

At the international workshop, I spoke on my nonhuman primate trials that had led me to propose testing DNA prime-MVA boost and MVA prime-MVA boost regimens for immunizations. Two CDC delegates, Tim Mastro and Sal Butera, reported on our AG vaccine, made with sequences that represented the dominant epidemic in the Ivory Coast. By the end of the workshop, the participants not only knew about our AG vaccine, but were enthusiastic about the potential for our vaccine to provide the much-needed vaccine for West Africa. Nkengasong and Mastro, two outstandingly capable men, who had a history of working together, would lead the vaccine into clinical trials as a collaboration between Projet RETRO-CI, the Ivorian Ministry of Health, the CDC and GeoVax.

The last day of our visit was sightseeing. The US embassy provided a car and a driver. We shopped at the main city bazaar, a maze of stalls with sellers hocking their wares. For myself, I purchased a set of "hear no evil, see no evil, say no evil" monkeys carved from ebony. For the members of the lab, I chose colorful tablecloths, fabric suitcases, and aprons. The driver then drove us out of town where we passed through densely packed suburbs with dirt paths between rows of simple single-story houses and then past vast acres of cocoa plantations (the Ivory Coast is the biggest cocoa producer in the world). Finally, the driver took us to beautiful white sand beaches. However, when I got out to walk, I found the beaches, which no one was using, fouled with crude oil hidden beneath the sand. The oil was nearly impossible to avoid and once stepped in, completely impossible to get off one's shoes.

The next joint meeting between the Ivoirians and the CDC would take place in September 2001, in Atlanta. On September 11, while we were meeting in the Yerkes conference room, my administrator burst in with the news that a jetliner had hit one of the twin towers of the World Trade Center in New York City. The 9/11 airline hijackings were taking place. It was a tragedy that unfolded over and dampened but did not stop planning for moving toward a trial of the AG vaccine.

The next planning session between the CDC and the Ivoirians would be in the Ivory Coast in January 2002. By this time, Simone Gbagbo, the First Lady of Ivory Coast, was supporting testing the AG vaccine. She had begun to attend meetings of the group and her entourage visited Emory and the CDC in February 2002.

A second international workshop on HIV/AIDS vaccines in the Côte d'Ivoire: "The National Vaccine Plan," was scheduled for September 2002. Nkengasong would speak in the opening session on "An HIV Vaccine for Africa—Introducing the African AIDS Vaccine Program," and Mastro would speak in the closing session on "Building Successful International HIV Vaccine Research Collaborations." Both Dennis Ellenberger (from the CDC) and I would speak on the AG DNA/MVA vaccine. The title of my talk was "Recent Advances in DNA-MVA Vaccines and Timelines for Phase 1 Trials in Côte d'Ivoire." Jeff Lennox, a new addition to our team from Emory, would speak on "Working with a Community Advisory Board in HIV Vaccine Trials." The closing remarks would be by First Lady Simone Gbagbo. We were making excellent progress toward testing the much-needed AG vaccine.

I arrived in Abidjan on the eve of the meeting. Driving to the hotel at dusk, I was surprised to see stacked tires partially barricading roads both into and within Abidjan. It was a little disconcerting. I checked into the Hotel Ivoire and visited the conference room, decked with red floral arrangements in preparation for the meeting. My room, on the sixth floor, had a view over the city.

Tired from the overseas flight, I went to bed only to be startled by what sounded like trucks crashing into concrete walls intermixed with loud popping. As I surfaced from sleep, it dawned on me that the noise was artillery and gunfire. I wasn't sure what to do. I kept my lights off, checked my door was double-locked, got dressed, looked for where to hide, tested whether I fit under my bed, and stayed away from my window. As the sun rose, I could see smoke rising from the city. I turned on my TV and saw the same view of smoke pluming over Abidjan—whoever was filming, was filming from the Hotel Ivoire. About 6:00 a.m. the leader of the CDC group, Alan Greenberg, called and said that there had been an attempted coup, that Abidjan was still in the hands of the government, that a twenty-four-hour curfew had been put in place, and that I could move around the hotel but should not go outside the hotel. The workshop was cancelled.

Looking out my window, I could not see a single person, just the billowing smoke. Not having heard gunfire for several hours, I went downstairs only to be shocked to find that the main door of the hotel had been shot through and the corridor of the first floor sprayed with bullets. Except for an Air France flight crew, and a Russian travel agent, the US participants for the cancelled workshop appeared to be the only guests in the hotel.

We met for dinner in the hotel dining room where we ate what remained to be eaten, talked, and then retired to bed. The next morning a life-size mannequin of a flight attendant, positioned by the front desk, held a notice: AIRPORT SHUTTLE, 10:00 A.M. I immediately got my suitcase and positioned myself next to the mannequin. There was no way that I was not going to be on that shuttle. We kept low in the shuttle as it drove through deserted streets to the airport. At the airport, the Air France flight that normally leaves at midnight for Paris was en route to pick us up. Meanwhile, the CDC members of our party, frazzled by having to get their passports from the safe at Projet RETRO-CI using a car with an "empty" gas tank, appeared and checked in. We were all looking for food, which was scarce because none of the food shops had opened.

An Airbus, Air France's largest passenger plane, appeared on the horizon. The plane touched down just long enough for us to board. It then flew to Togo to refuel and provision for the flight to Paris. It was such a relief to be in the air, leaving the burning tires and scattered gunfire behind. The next morning as I looked for the gate for my connecting flight to Atlanta, my heart leapt when through the concourse windows I saw the signature tail of a Delta airliner. I was going home! I boarded the plane with tears in my eyes.

The attempted coup would mark the beginning of several years of civil war. The Gbagbos would be voted out of power and arrested when they refused to yield power. A country that had been one of the most stable in Africa was no longer suitable for conducting clinical trials. Our most promising and fastest hare was down and out.

At this point plans for what would prove to be the tortoise—clinical trials for the clade B vaccine—were plodding through the US HVTN, the NIH Division of AIDS, and the FDA, while plans for trials for the clade C vaccine were undergoing intermittent spurts, interspersed with voluminous paperwork.

Testing the Clade C Vaccine in India, 2001–2005

Contacts for testing the clade C vaccine in India came through Rafi Ahmed, the Director of the Emory Vaccine Center. Ahmed, a member of an advisory board for India's Department of Biotechnology, was an active consultant on limiting the spread of HIV in India. Given the public health threat of AIDS, the Secretary of the Department of Biotechnology, Manju Sharma, invited Ahmed and GeoVax to present our clade C vaccine to Indian leaders in virology and biotechnology. Ahmed, Hildebrand (CEO of GeoVax), Rama Rao Amara (an exceptionally capable research fellow from India), and I flew to Delhi in December 2001 to meet with Varaprasad Reddy, the CEO of Shantha Biotechnics, and Shahid Jameel, an academic virologist. Shantha Biotechnics was successfully manufacturing an affordable hepatitis B virus vaccine for India. Jameel was establishing a virology program at the new International Center for Biotechnology and Genetics. Over the next several months, a return visit to India was made by Hildebrand and Amara to visit Shantha Biotechnics. This visit was followed by Reddy, the CEO and founder of Shantha, coming to Atlanta to visit GeoVax and the Emory Vaccine Center. On a separate trip, Amara and I visited the National AIDS Research Institute in Pune, the institute that had been mandated to conduct HIV clinical trials.

These visits, along with leadership provided by Peggy Johnston of the US NIH Division of AIDS, activated a dormant Vaccine Action Program that had been formed to fund joint projects between American and Indian scientists. In 2005, we successfully secured a joint project. However, most of the available dollars in the program were Indian and could not go outside of India. Rather than funding the clade C vaccine, the award ended up being used to fund Jameel's new virology program at the International Center for Genetics and Biotechnology. Our second hare had fallen out of the race.

Despite the Vaccine Action Program not leading to clinical trials, multiple visits to India did open a new world for me. The offices of the Department of Biotechnology, Indian government offices, were guarded by exceptionally handsome and tall Indians in dress military uniform. One felt important when one checked in. Meeting rooms had pictures of Gandhi. Outside, many streets and sidewalks were not paved. In Pune, where our driver stopped at the local bus terminal to get directions to the National AIDS Research Institute, the buses were in hubcap-deep mud. There were animals, especially cows, everywhere. One of my favorite memories is a half dozen cows lined up on a center strip, all facing the same way, into traffic. When one took the road to the Taj Mahal, modern two- to four-story industrial buildings flanked a highway used by cars, elephants, donkeys, and people. The Golden Quadrilateral, a new and first national highway, was being built by hand-splitting rocks the size of cantaloupes, to rocks the size of avocadoes that were in turn chipped by a series of workers to increasingly smaller sizes, ending in gravel. The gravel was then carried by women using woven baskets on their heads to a growing roadbed. City soundscapes were a symphony. Cars with different toned horns beeped once to pass, and then twice, once passed: beep, beep/beep. Vans had a driver and a helper, who opened and closed the van door and gave hand signals for left-hand turns. Red traffic lights in Delhi displayed the word, RELAX. The food was exotic, although I had to be careful to only eat recently cooked, and still physically hot, food. A former student who had returned to India, told me that the only sure way to not get diarrhea was to eat hard-boiled eggs that I had peeled myself and to drink lassis, a wonderful yogurt-like drink.

Looking back, I can see that the failure to get HIV vaccine trials underway was a greater missed opportunity for the Ivory Coast than for India. In the early 2000s, a major difference between the two countries was the incidence of AIDS. In the Ivory Coast the incidence of HIV was approximately 10 percent. In contrast, the rate in India was <1 percent. HIV was a much greater health priority for the Ivory Coast than for India. Also, the Ivory Coast had prepared for trials and established infrastructure (Projet RETRO-CI) and cohorts for running preventative HIV trials. Such infrastructure and cohorts had not been established in India. The Ivory Coast also benefitted from the ability of Nkengasong and Mastro, working together, to get things done. They were not just trying to get money for their institutes. They were actively conducting clinical trials, working to curtail a devastating pandemic. It is a tragedy that an HIV vaccine program, which had held so much promise, had been interrupted by civil unrest in the Ivory Coast.

Testing the Clade B Vaccine in the Americas, 2001–2019

Trials of the GeoVax clade B HIV vaccine, the tortoise, would plod down the road over the next two decades. The clade B vaccine would be tested by the HVTN, a network of clinical sites at academic institutions formed by the NIH in 2000 to test candidate AIDS vaccines. Between 2001 and 2017, the HVTN would conduct five early-stage trials testing different regimens of the GeoVax DNA and MVA vaccines for safety and vaccine responses. Each of these trials would be initiated by submitting a vaccine concept to the HVTN leadership committee. Once the concept was approved, an overview of the proposed protocol would be submitted to the Division of AIDS protocol committee where it would undergo review and response. If approved by the Division of AIDS protocol committee, the HVTN leadership would assign a protocol chair, a protocol co-chair, a protocol team leader, a statistician, a medical officer, and trial sites to develop the full protocol and the informed consent form that participants would sign before receiving inoculations. These documents were at least a hundred pages of single-space typing.

In parallel with the development of the protocol, the candidate vaccine would undergo manufacture, release and toxicity testing under GMP/GLP conditions. Regulatory filings to support testing of the vaccine would be submitted to the FDA by the NIH Division of AIDS. The most important regulatory filing was the Investigational New Drug (IND) application. The FDA facilitated IND fillings by holding pre-IND meetings. For a pre-IND meeting, GeoVax would prepare and the Division of AIDS would review and submit a meeting request. A briefing package for the IND would be due within thirty days of the meeting request, and the pre-IND meeting would take place a further thirty days later. The pre-IND meetings, which afforded a review of the proposed vaccine candidate, its proposed manufacture, release and toxicity testing, and the proposed protocol for clinical testing, were extremely helpful as they guided the development of the vaccine and its IND. When the vaccines and protocol were ready, the Division of AIDS would submit and maintain the IND. Following the receipt of an application for an IND, the FDA would have thirty days to review the package and allow the proposed trial to proceed or to put the proposed trial on hold.

GeoVax's roles in the trials were to supply clinical product to the Division of AIDS pharmacy for distribution to the trial sites, to provide an investigator's brochure on the characteristics and testing of the candidate vaccines, (typically a fifty-to-sixty-page single-spaced document) and to prepare and appropriately update the chemistry, manufacturing, and controls sections of the IND for the vaccine products. Once all was in place, trial sites would be reviewed by the HVTN and Division of AIDS and the site personnel trained on the trial protocol. The trial would then start.

The clade B vaccine plodded down the road not only because of the time it took HVTN and the Division of AIDS committees to review concepts and protocols but also because

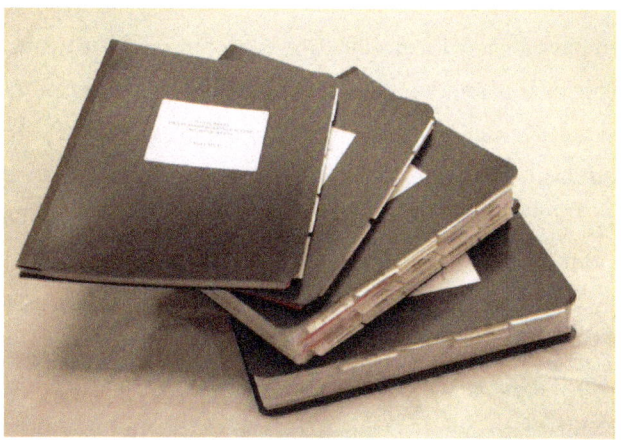

IND for HVTN 045. Our first, and shortest, IND for our first, and simplest trial (HVTN 045). This trial tested only the DNA vaccine.

the academic trial sites turned out to be slow to enroll, many enrolling less than one participant per month. In my eyes, this reflected the trial sites liking the support they received from the HVTN to help run their clinics. This resulted in the clinics not feeling any urgency to get the trials done. Contrary to popular expectations, I found the FDA reviews both efficient and knowledgeable. The reviews in the NIH Division of AIDS were more idiosyncratic. This staff did not have the broad experience with clinical trials that the FDA staff benefited from. I learned to be at the NIH for Division of AIDS reviews to be able to respond to concerns as they arose.

All of the GeoVax HVTN trials would be placebo-controlled double-blind trials in which neither the recipient nor the health care worker who delivered an inoculation knew whether the recipient was receiving vaccine or placebo. Safety findings were monitored by the Division of AIDS safety review team, which was available twenty-four hours a day, seven days a week for notification of potential life-threatening adverse events and which met weekly to review routine safety and reactogenicity data for ongoing Division of AIDS trials. Throughout the trials, blood would be harvested for analyses for raised immune responses conducted by HVTN Central Laboratories. All data would be entered into a central database at HVTN headquarters in Seattle where it would be analyzed by HVTN statisticians.

GeoVax staff and I would participate in closed-session protocol team meetings at the spring and fall HVTN Full Group meetings and draft annual reports, including updated chemistry, manufacturing and controls information. The Division of AIDS would review and submit this information to the FDA. I would also help the protocol chair with the sections of manuscripts relevant to the GeoVax products. In all, the HVTN would conduct five clinical trials involving about five hundred volunteers on the clade B GeoVax products.

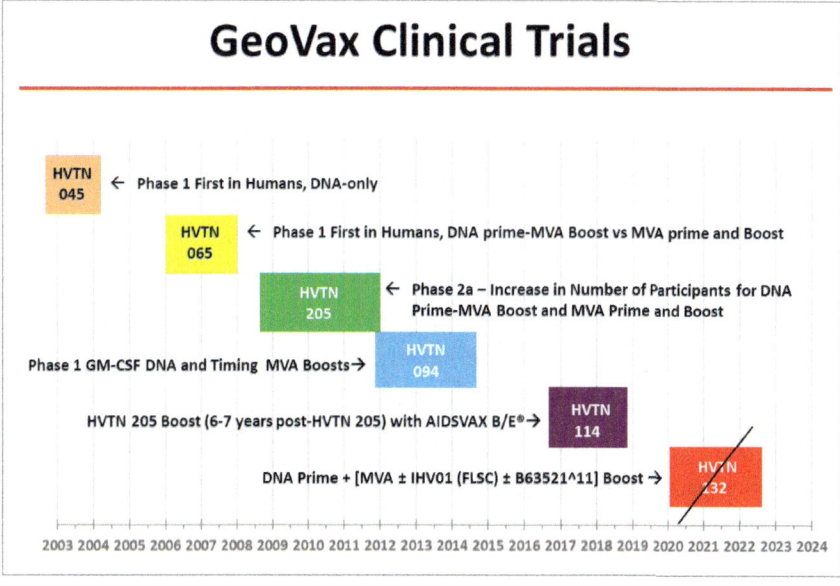

Overview of Clinical Trials. Trials were conducted on the GeoVax clade B DNA and MVA Vaccines by the HVTN. Trial numbers are designated in colored boxes. The phase and purpose of the trials are stated beside trial boxes. The timeline for the trials is at the bottom of the Figure. The line through Trial HVTN 132 indicates that this trial was abandoned due to the pressing need to test COVID vaccines. The timelines are adapted from a schematic prepared by the Division of AIDS

HVTN 045: 2003–2005 (30 participants)

HVTN 045, our first Phase 1 trial, was a dose escalation study of the clade B DNA vaccine. The HVTN 045 trial showed that the highest practical dose of DNA was well tolerated with no serious adverse events. Tests for elicited immune responses revealed that the DNA had raised very low, if even detectable, antibody and T cell responses.

HVTN 065: 2006–2008 (120 participants)

The next Phase 1 trial tested the clade B DNA prime with the clade B MVA boost and clade B MVA priming and boosting. The DNA prime-MVA boost protocol was tested because of the strong immune responses that this regimen had elicited in nonhuman primates. For this first-in-human combination, one-tenth doses of the DNA and MVA vaccines were tested in a ten-participant group before testing full doses of the DNA and MVA vaccines in three groups of thirty-participants testing no, one, and two DNA primes for an MVA boost. All three of the full dose regimens were well tolerated with no serious adverse events. Immunogenicity data from the Central Laboratories showed that the DNA prime-MVA boost regimens elicited the highest levels of antiviral white blood cells whereas MVA inoculations, in the absence of a DNA prime, elicited the highest levels of antibody to Env.

As the HVTN tested vaccines in its network, it compared the heights and breadths of immune responses elicited by different vaccines. The underlying assumption was that vaccines raising the most robust responses would have the best chance at providing protection. The GeoVax HVTN 065 trial was the sixty-fifth Phase 1 trial that the HVTN had conducted. At the 2008 fall HVTN Meeting, the results of recently completed Phase 1 trials were presented. Except for results obtained for the poxvirus-vectored vaccines of Therion Inc., our vaccines had raised the most robust antibody and T cell responses. Therion had gone out of business due to the failure of its cancer program. GeoVax, with the vaccine designs we had honed in monkey and lab studies, was still standing.

Our GeoVax vaccine also distinguished itself from other vaccines in eliciting both anti-HIV white blood cells and anti-HIV antibody. The first vaccines into efficacy trials had focused on eliciting anti-Env antibody or antiviral white blood cells, not both. VaxGen Inc. had tested bivalent gp120 proteins for the ability to raise protective antibody in intravenous drug users in Thailand (VAX 003 trial) and in couples in which one member was HIV positive and the other HIV negative in the United States (VAX 004 trial). Merck had used adenoviral vectors to test a vaccine that raised anti-HIV white blood cells in men who have sex with men in the United States (STEP trial) and in heterosexual volunteers in South Africa (Phambili Trial). By the fall of 2008, both these approaches had failed to provide protection in efficacy trials.

HVTN 205: 2009 –2012 (299 participants)

HVTN 205, a Phase 2a trial, would have a total pf 299 participants that would test three regimens. The first, the DNA-MVA regimen, would test injections of two full doses of DNA at months 0 and 2 followed by injections of two full doses of MVA at months 4 and 6. In the second regimen, the MVA-only regimen, participants would receive full doses of MVA at months 0, 2 and 6. The third regimen, the placebo group, would receive placebo at months 0, 2, 4, and 6.

The HVTN 205 trial was in low-risk individuals with ten trial sites in the United States and two trial sites in Peru. As in HVTN 045 and HVTN 065, no severe adverse events related to the vaccine were observed. Encouragingly, at peak responses, 93.2 percent of the DNA-MVA group and 98.4 percent of the MVA-only group scored with anti-Env antibody. As in the smaller Phase 1 HVTN 065 trial, responses for antiviral white blood cells were higher in the DNA-MVA group than in the

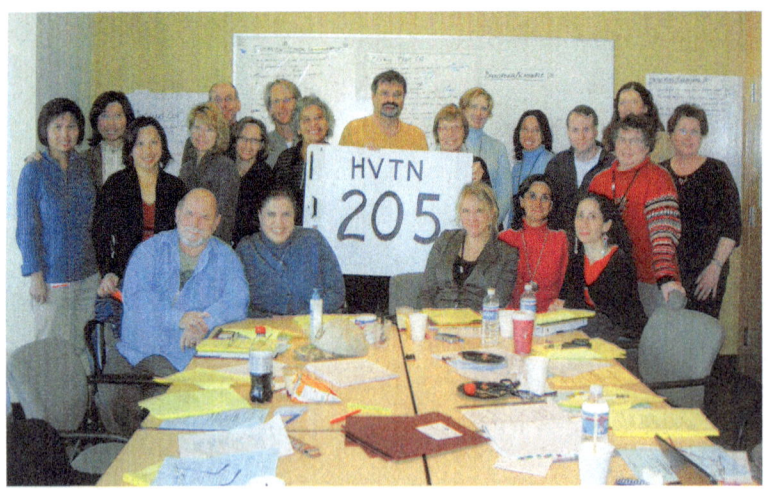

The HVTN 205 Protocol Team. This team picture was taken during a two-day face-to-face meeting preparing the HVTN 205 trial protocol. Massimo Cardinali, our NIH Medical Officer, is holding the HVTN 205 banner. Facing the picture, I am immediately to the right of Massimo. Paul Goepfert, Protocol Chair, and Carter Bentley, Protocol Development Coordinator, are to the left of Massimo in the back row. The protocol team leader, Marnie Elizaga, is the most left-hand person in the middle row. Huguette Redinger, the most right-hand person in the back row was project manager.

MVA-only group, whereas elicited antibody was higher in the MVA-only group. Also encouragingly, at six months after vaccination, the levels of the elicited antibody and white blood cells had decreased by less than threefold in both the DNA-MVA and MVA-only groups. The GeoVax vaccines had raised remarkably durable immune responses. This is likely due to MVA, an attenuated smallpox vaccine, having retained the ability of its smallpox parent to raise durable vaccine responses.

Two Additional Phase 1 Trials, 2012–2020

In 2012, following the completion of HVTN 205, GeoVax sought to go on to a Phase 2b trial in an at-risk population to determine whether the vaccine might provide evidence for protection and merit going forward to an efficacy trial. The HVTN dragged its heels over concerns that GeoVax might go under, like some other small companies. The HVTN also was concerned that we did not have as high immune responses as elicited by the best vaccines for raising just antibody or just anti-HIV white blood cells. So instead of proceeding to Phase 2b testing, the HVTN took our vaccine into two additional Phase 1 trials to explore conditions that might increase the height and breadth of elicited antibody responses to Env. It was very disappointing for both us and our investors to not be going forward into a 2b trial.

The first additional Phase 1 trial (HVTN 094) (2012–2015) (48 participants) used a novel DNA prime that co-expressed granulocyte-macrophage colony-stimulating factor (GM-CSF) along with HIV virus-like particles. GM-CSF is a protein that attracts white blood cells to the site of an infection, or in our case, the site of vaccination. In studies in nonhuman primates, the co-expression of GM-CSF in the GeoVax SIV vaccine had increased the level of protection from 25 percent to 71 percent. This increase in protection had correlated with an increase in avidity (the tightness of binding) of the elicited antibody to Env. Given these results we undertook a larger macaque trial to test the reproducibility of the effects of co-expressed GM-CSF on the protection elicited by our SIV vaccine. At the same time, the HVTN undertook HVTN 094, a Phase 1 trial in humans to test whether co-expressed GM-CSF would enhance the strength of binding of the elicited antibody to Env. The HVTN 094 trial also tested the effects of a third MVA boost and greater spacing between boosts (four months as opposed to two months) on the height and tightness of the binding of elicited antibody to Env.

Disappointingly, the trial in nonhuman primates did not repeat the results of the first trial: protection was not enhanced by co-expressing GM-CSF with the DNA prime. However, the results of HVTN 094, conducted in humans, showed that an additional boost and longer spacing of immunization between boosts increased antibody responses. However, HVTN 094 did not show an effect of co-expressed GM-CSF on the binding characteristics of antibody responses. Given these results, co-expressed GM-CSF, was not taken forward, whereas an additional MVA boost, spaced with a 4-month interval between boosts, was planned for future trials.

The second additional Phase 1 trial (HVTN 114) (27 participants) tested the ability of a gp120 protein boost to enhance antibody responses elicited by the GeoVax DNA-MVA and MVA-MVA vaccines. We had tested adding a gp120 protein boost to our MVA boost in the SHIV-macaque model in 2001-2002 and found that the protein boost increased the levels of elicited antibody by more than tenfold. However, the high level of elicited antibody had appeared to decrease, rather than increase, protection. We had attributed the decrease in protection to gp120, a subunit of Env, failing to elicit effective antibody against the natural form of Env.

Meanwhile, a vaccine which the HVTN had considered too weak to take into Phase 3 testing had been taken forward as part of a long-term collaboration between the US military and the Thailand Ministry of Public Health (the Thais). This vaccine, a "pox-protein" vaccine, combined two vaccines that had failed in earlier trials: a canarypox vaccine developed by Sanofi-Pasteur and a bivalent (two component) gp120 protein vaccine developed by VaxGen Inc. The US military and the Thai Department of Public Health conducted a Phase 3 trial in which the canarypox vaccine was inoculated at months 0, 1, 3, and 6 and the bivalent gp120 protein vaccine was co-inoculated with the canarypox vaccine at months 3 and 6. Both the pox and protein vaccines had been matched to the predominant viruses in the Thai epidemic. Unexpectedly, the trial, a community trial, conducted in 16,402 mostly heterosexual men, achieved 31.2 percent protection. The US military and the Thais reported these results on September 24, 2009, in Paris where the US military (in full dress uniform) proudly reported they had "kicked the door in" for making an HIV vaccine. The field was electrified by finally having a success, albeit a very modest success and a success that has since failed to repeat.

The Thai trial impacted our vaccine program by stimulating the HVTN to test the ability of the same gp120 protein that had been used in the Thai trial to boost antibody elicited by the GeoVax DNA-MVA and MVA-MVA vaccines. This trial was designated HVTN 114 and conducted from 2017 to 2020. To expedite the testing of the gp120 boost of GeoVax's vaccine, the HVTN conducted HVTN 114 in participants from our earlier HVTN 205 trial. Twenty-seven (out of 299) participants in HVTN 205 were located who were willing to test a gp120 protein boost. The twenty-seven previously immunized volunteers were boosted with either the MVA vaccine, the gp120 protein vaccine, or both vaccines. By the time the HVTN 114 trial was initiated in 2017, a median of seven years had lapsed after the last inoculation in the original HVTN 205 trial. Despite this long "rest," antibody responses to HIV could be detected in sera harvested prior to the boost in 62 percent of the participants. Further evidence of HVTN 205 having raised long-lasting responses was shown by every single one of the twenty-seven participants undergoing strong post boost memory expansions of antibody responses to HIV gp120.

These responses to gp120 were much higher than the responses that had been obtained in HVTN 205 and included responses to the V1V2 subregion of gp120 that had correlated with protection in the "successful" Thai trial. Given the large increases in antibody responses with the gp120 protein boost, the NIH Division of AIDS initiated manufacture of gp120 proteins representing recent patient isolates to test gp120 protein boosting of the GeoVax DNA-MVA and MVA-MVA vaccines.

The HVTN leadership assigned a protocol team to plan HVTN 132, a Phase 1 trial to test the ability of the newly manufactured gp120 proteins to boost the gp120 antibody elicited by the GeoVax clade B DNA-MVA and MVA-MVA vaccines. But then, in 2020, planning for the trial was stopped by the emergence of the SARS-CoV2 pandemic and the urgent need for the NIH supported clinical trial networks to test candidate vaccines for COVID-19.

I was deeply disappointed to see our work come to a stuttering halt, given the years of work that we had put into the GeoVax vaccine. However, of the ten currently completed efficacy trials for HIV vaccines, only one, the Thai trial, has achieved even some success (a 31.2 percent reduction in infection). HIV may be an infection that is so adept at hiding from the immune system that a vaccine is impossible. Encouragingly, drugs are proving to be highly effective at both controlling and preventing HIV infections. So given increasingly effective drugs, NIH funds, which were supporting the HIV vaccine effort, may better be directed toward drug delivery, a highly promising area of HIV control and prevention.

Looking back at our effort to develop an HIV vaccine, where could we have been more effective? Our major limitation was money. If we had had sufficient funding, we could have set the pace and focus of early phase clinical testing rather than being dependent on HVTN and Division of AIDS committees to advance our vaccine. By not having sufficient funds we were dependent on decisions by ever-changing "experts" to advance the testing of the GeoVax vaccine. After our Phase 2a HVTN 205 trial we should have gone on to a Phase 2b trial in at risk individuals. If this had shown evidence of possible protection, we then could have gone on to a Phase 3 efficacy trial. If this trial had not shown protection, the program would have arrived at a natural termination.

The abandonment of the GeoVax DNA-MVA and MVA-MVA HIV vaccines by the HVTN and Division of AIDS meant that GeoVax would be losing what had been its signature product. But in its twenty-one years of existence, GeoVax has moved from being a private, single-product company to a shareholder's multi-product company. Two Phase 2 trials for COVID-19 had already supplanted the once premier position of HIV in the company's pipeline. MVA vaccine technology had supplanted the original dominance of the DNA vaccine technology. However, the expression of noninfectious virus-like particles, displaying target antigens for immunization, remains a mantra for the company's approach to vaccine development. These target antigens have expanded from the HIV Env protein to the spike (envelope) proteins of Zika, COVID-19, Ebola, Marburg, and Sudan hemorrhagic fever viruses and a cancer antigen. As of 2024, GeoVax continues its work on developing "Vaccines Serving Humanity."

Epilogue: 2024

As for me, I am enjoying life outside of the lab. My son Bill, now a chaired professor at Stanford, gave a talk at the Vi, a Continuing Care Community on the Stanford campus. He was sufficiently impressed that he called and said "Mom, there is a place for retirees on the Stanford campus. It is not like an old folk's home. People live in independent units until they need more care. You should join." I now very happily live at the Vi. enjoying the dinnertime conversations, helping with the Current Events lecture series, taking exercise classes, walking the neighborhood, and hiking the coastal hills.

So, was it hard to leave a career in science? I had ridden four waves of exciting science. My PhD thesis contributed to early studies on messenger RNA by defining the range of sizes and the timing of messenger RNA movement from its synthesis in the nucleus to the protein synthetic machinery in the cytoplasm. On the second wave I contributed to the discovery of proto-oncogenes and the demonstration that retroviruses could cause cancer by proviral insertions mutating proto-oncogenes to oncogenes. On the third wave, which grew from my work with retroviruses, I pioneered the use of DNA for vaccines. These studies set foundations for the current highly successful messenger RNA (mRNA) vaccines. My last wave was cofounding GeoVax and taking DNA-MVA and MVA-MVA vaccines for HIV into early-stage trials in humans.

On my leaving science, Yerkes, Emory and GeoVax all roasted me at farewell events. The HVTN gave me the Gita Ramjee Award "in appreciation of outstanding commitment and contributions to HIV prevention research." I had loved my career, but I had made my contributions and have turned down opportunities to review programs and serve on committees. I made many friendships over the decades of my work in science. I marvel as I watch the careers of my students, fellows, and employees.

In the beginning, I was born into a productive and happy family. I have now come full circle, back to family life. Against the background of my life at the Vi, I am the grandma who gets to applaud at school plays, admire the young lacrosse players, talk politics and climate change with the college students. I am no longer lead chef at family events, but I enjoy my role as a sous-chef. I was blessed with an exciting and fruitful career, but now am blessed with the continuing warmth, wonder, and adventure of my family and friends. At my 1967 arrival in Palo Alto, I had been in labor with Bill, my firstborn. On my return in 2017, fifty years later, Bill and Peggy, his wife, would care for me.

I have had a wonderful life, far exceeding what I ever could have anticipated as a young girl nervously visiting a Radcliffe dean, seeking to take courses in science instead of courses in education. This dean not only let me know that I, a girl, could be a scientist but encouraged me to become a scientist. Along the way, I have had the adventure of Moscow, the romance of a man I loved who truly loved me, the marvel of babies, the joy of successful sons and last, but not least, the exhilaration of a career in molecular biology.

Acknowledgments

I would like to thank my parents, Ruth Nichols and Allen Latham Jr., for giving me the confidence and curiosity to explore the worlds that opened for me throughout my life. I am particularly indebted to my father for his love and his ability to see positive and productive solutions for virtually any predicament.

I am indebted to my MIT thesis advisor, James E. Darnell Jr., for taking me on as his first graduate student. His quantitative approach to research coupled with his insistence on showing raw, not just normalized, data remain with me to this day. I also wish to acknowledge Thomas R. Insel, the former Director of the Yerkes Primate Research Center who hired me at the age of sixty to be the Chief of Microbiology and Immunology. Insel made possible a rich last chapter for my academic life.

I am indebted to the Chief Economic Officers of GeoVax, Inc.: Don Hildebrand, Bob McNally, and David Dodd, who oversaw the business side of the company I cofounded with Hildebrand to help take my HIV vaccine into human trials.

I am forever indebted to my students, fellows, technical staff, and sabbatical professors who provided both hands and intellect for the research in my academic and GeoVax labs. Daily life in the lab was a rich mix of their insights, activities, and personalities as we moved down the field toward our goals. I thank the administrative staff, both academic and company, who managed schedules, fielded calls and compiled the grants that helped fund my research. I salute and thank all of you for enabling and enriching my life.

Over the years, especially as I reentered science following my time out to raise the boys to school age, I have collaborated with scientists and labs that had expertise that complemented my expertise and resources. This was particularly true in the years where I bred chickens for endogenous retroviruses and contributed to studies showing that retroviruses could cause cancer by insertional mutagenesis. I am deeply indebted to both those named as well as those not named for these collaborations.

And finally, I am indebted to Ed Schein, my late-in-life companion; Amy L. Bernstein, my book coach, Maria Latham, Paul Rosa, Kathy Lachenauer, Carol Ude and my sons, who encouraged me in my writing and offered critical comments as my autobiography emerged.

Glossary of Terms

adjuvant: A substance that enhances the body's immune response.

antibody: Y-shaped immunoglobulins (proteins) that bind to antigens. Antibodies can bind to an infectious agent (for example a viral spike protein) blocking its ability to infect.

antigen: Any substance that upon injection into a vertebrate is capable of eliciting the production of antibody.

avian myelocytomatosis virus: Retrovirus that has incorporated sequences from the cellular myc proto-oncogene into its genome. The *myc* expressing virus causes a white blood cell cancer in chickens.

base: Nucleotide components of DNA and RNA polymers that include adenine, thymine (or uracil in RNA), cytosine and guanine.

base-pairing rules: The requirement that adenine must always form a base-pair with thymine (or uracil) and guanine with cytosine during the copying of a nucleic acid.

Biosafety Level: A set of precautions required to work with pathogens in a laboratory. The levels of containment range from the lowest (Biosafety Level 1) to the highest (Biosafety Level 4). Most work is done at Biosafety Level 2

bursa of Fabricius: In birds, the bursa of Fabricius is an outpocketing of the gut where white blood cells that become antibody-producing B cells undergo development.

cancer: A disease in which cells grow uncontrollably and spread throughout the body.

carcinogen: A substance or physical condition that predisposes a vertebrate for the development of cancer.

CD4 T cells: The type of white blood cell that provides help in the form of growth factors for other white blood cells. CD4 is the receptor for human immunodeficiency virus and CD4 T cells (also called helper cells) are the target cells for HIV infection. In contrast to CD4 T cells, CD8 T cells are killer T cells (see cytotoxic T cells, below).

CDC: Centers for Disease Control and Prevention, the federal bureau that protects the public health of US citizens.

CEO: Chief Economic Officer.

challenge infection: A planned infection to test whether a vaccine or drug is providing protection.

clades: Genetically distinct versions of a virus. For HIV, clades are generally about 20 percent different in their sequence from each other.

cloaca: Single posterior opening for avian digestive, urinary, and reproductive tracts.

clone: Exact genetic copies of a DNA sequence.

c-myc: Proto-oncogene that was incorporated into avian myelocytomatosis virus where it is an oncogene.

Communion: A Christian sacrament in which bread and wine are remembrances of Jesus' sacrifice on the cross.

cytoplasm: The nonnuclear portion of a cell.

cytotoxic T cells: White blood cells that recognize and kill pathogen infected cells.

DNA: Deoxyribonucleic acid, double helical polymers of deoxyribonucleotide bases (adenine, thymine, guanine and cytosine) that follow base-pairing rules (adenine with thymine and guanine with cytosine) that provide the heritable genetic code for life.

DNA vaccine: A vaccine that expresses the immunizing antigen in a DNA expression vector that is directly inoculated into a vertebrate.

DNA-MVA vaccine: A vaccine that consists of priming with a DNA vaccine and then boosting with a MVA vaccine.

endogenous virus: A virus that has become inserted into

germline DNA and is being transmitted in the DNA of eggs and sperm. Endogenous viruses make up a substantial fraction of the DNA of vertebrates.

Env: A generic designation for the glycoproteins on the membranes of retroviruses that mediate entry into cells.

enzyme: Molecules (proteins or RNA) capable of accelerating (catalyzing) chemical reactions.

exogenous virus: A virus that is spreading as an infection in contrast to endogenous viruses that are transmitted in the DNA of eggs and sperm. Exogenous viruses can be benign or pathogenic.

express: Produce the protein encoded in an RNA or DNA, expression vectors are designed to produce encoded proteins.

FDA: Food and Drug Administration, agency that oversees human and veterinary products in the United States, products regulated by the FDA include food, drugs, and medical devices.

filtrate: Portion of a mixture of substances that can pass through a filter. Most filters involve pore sizes. However filters can also include chemicals that bond agents undergoing filtration.

fowl pox vector: Use of fowl pox virus (a member of the same family of viruses as smallpox) to carry foreign genes into cells.

gene: DNA sequence that encodes a messenger RNA for a functional protein.

gp120: A monomer of the receptor binding subunit of the gp160 Envelope glycoprotein of HIV.

gp140: A secreted monomer of the gp160 Env protein of HIV, that includes the gp120 receptor binding subunit and the extracellular region of the transmembrane subunit of Env.

gp160: A monomer of the gp120 receptor binding and transmembrane protein of Env. The native Env protein is a trimer comprising three copies of gp160.

HIV: Human immunodeficiency virus, a pathogenic retrovirus of humans that has killed more than forty million people.

humoral: Antibody responses found in blood.

HVTN: HIV Vaccine Trials Network is a US funded and led international collaboration formed to test candidate HIV vaccines.

IND: Investigational New Drug application reviewed by the FDA before a biologic is allowed to be tested in humans.

insertional mutagenesis: The insertion of a DNA sequence into chromosomal DNA that mutates the expression of the recipient DNA.

integration: The insertion of a foreign DNA into the genome (DNA) of a vertebrate host.

isolate: A pathogen that has been recovered from a diseased host. Each recovery is a separate isolate.

laboratory-adapted: An isolate of a pathogen that has been serially passaged (grown) under laboratory conditions. The serial growth selects mutations that support growth under laboratory conditions.

life cycle: The steps a pathogen goes through to replicate itself. For example a retrovirus life cycle involves entry followed by reverse transcription of RNA to DNA followed by integration of the newly synthesized DNA to form a provirus followed by expression of the proteins encoded in the provirus and the assembly and budding of mature virus from the infected cell.

liposome: Liposomes are small vesicles in which lipids encapsulate substances to be delivered to cells.

lymphoma: A cancer of white blood cells.

memory: Immune responses have acute and memory phases. In the acute phase the subset of white blood cells that recognize an invading pathogen expands to fight the infection. Once an infection is controlled, long-lived memory cells are formed that patrol the body. These memory cells undergo rapid mobilization should the infection reappear and are the basis for vaccine responses.

messenger RNA (mRNA): RNA that determines what DNA will be translated into protein and serves as a template for protein synthesis.

molecular biology: The study of biological molecules and their interactions that create life.

MVA: Modified Vaccinia Ankara, an attenuated form of the smallpox vaccine that is used as a safer smallpox vaccine and as a vector for vaccine development.

mutation: The change of a DNA sequence so that it no longer codes for its original activity.

myelocytomatosis: A white blood cell cancer.

naked DNA: Purified DNA that is being delivered to cells without liposome encapsulation.

neutralizing antibody: The subset of antibodies that block an infection. Most neutralizing antibodies act on viral proteins that mediate entry into cells.

NIAID: National Institute of Allergy and Infectious Diseases, an institute within the US Department of Health Services.

nucleotide: Compounds comprised of carbon, oxygen, hydrogen, and phosphate that form the individual bases of a DNA polymer.

nucleus: The central organelle in cells that contains the cell's DNA.

oncogene: A gene that causes cancer. Oncogenes are mutations of normal cellular genes (proto-oncogenes) that control growth and development of cells.

points to consider: Documents developed by the US FDA to provide guidance on the manufacture and use of agents being developed for human or veterinary medicine.

polysome: Several ribosomes actively moving along and translating a mRNA.

Projet RETRO-CI: A former AIDS clinic established in Ivory Coast as a collaboration between the US CDC and the Ivoirian Ministry of Health.

promoter: DNA sequences that control the expression (production) of messenger RNAs.

protein: Strings (polymers) of amino acids translated from the genetic code in messenger RNAs. Each amino acid is coded for by three bases.

proto-oncogene: A gene that codes for normal growth and differentiation that can be mutated to cause cancer. Its cancer-causing form is termed an oncogene.

provirus: The DNA form of a retrovirus that has become inserted into the chromosomal DNA of its host.

recombinant: Linking of two DNAs to form a single DNA.

reverse transcriptase: An enzyme (protein) that copies (transcribes) RNA into DNA, the reverse of transcribing DNA to RNA.

ribosome: Small cellular particle that translates mRNA to proteins.

RNA: A polymer of ribonucleotide bases (adenine, thymine, guanine, and uracil).

Rous helper virus: Minimally pathogenic retroviruses of chickens that support the growth of Rous sarcoma virus by providing viral proteins that were lost when Rous sarcoma virus acquired the src oncogene. Rous helper viruses can cause cancer when proviral insertions convert a proto-oncogene to an oncogene or result in the incorporation of cellular proto-oncogene sequences into a virus to create a viral oncogene.

sarcoma: Tumor of muscle cells.

SHIV: Laboratory-constructed chimera of simian and human immunodeficiency virus.

SIV: Simian immunodeficiency virus, retroviruses that are endemic in nonhuman primates.

transcribe: A process in which the base pairs of DNA are used to order a complementary sequence of bases in RNA (see base-pairing rules).

U. Mass: The University of Massachusetts Medical School.

vector: A DNA plasmid, a virus, or a bacterium that has been engineered to carry a foreign DNA into cells.

virus: Infectious disease agent that requires host cells for replication. Viruses can contain DNA or RNA as their genetic information.

white blood cells: Blood cells provide a defense system for the body. White blood cells include T cells, B cells, monocytes, neutrophils, eosinophils, and basophils, all of which provide different defense functions. They are white because they do not contain the hemoglobin found in red blood cells that carry oxygen.

WHO: World Health Organization, located in Geneva, is an agency of the United Nations that coordinates global health policies.

Glossary of Key Contributors

Ahmed, Rafi: Director of the Emory Vaccine Center, expert on memory immune responses.

Astrin, Susan: Key collaborator on the characterization of endogenous avian leukosis viruses in normal chicken DNA.

Baltimore, David: Fellow in the Darnell lab when I was a graduate student, co-winner of the Nobel Prize for the discovery of reverse transcriptase.

Berg, Jack: Early employee at GeoVax who piloted production of DNA and MVA.

Butera, Sal: Scientist at CDC who helped with the development of the AG DNA vaccine.

Darnell, Jim: Thesis advisor at MIT and then after his move, at the Albert Einstein College of Medicine; pioneer in the study of mRNA and its expression.

Eagle, Harry: Chair of Department of Cell Biology at Albert Einstein College of Medicine, developed a defined medium for growing cultured cells.

Ellenberger, Dennis: Scientist at CDC who helped with the development of the AG DNA vaccine.

Ennis, Frank: Professor of Medicine at U. Mass who advised me to prepare a one-page memo re: my needs for monkeys for studies on SIV DNA vaccines.

Felgner, Phil: Developer of liposomes for delivery of DNA into cells.

Fenyo, Eva Maria: Swedish collaborator who provided molecularly cloned Envs from serial patient isolates.

Fuller, Deborah: Scientist, originally at Agracetus, who helped develop use of gene gun.

Fynan, Ellen: Postdoctoral fellow who played a major role in early DNA vaccine development, currently a professor of biology at Worcester State.

Gbagbo, Laurent and Simone: President and First Lady of the Ivory Coast who supported trials for the prevention of AIDS but were overthrown in a civil war.

Guillory, Espaze: Provided outstanding childcare for boys when they were pre-school.

Hale, Marion: Roommate in Boston for my first year at MIT, Hale is her maiden name.

Hanafusa, Hidesaburo: Scientist who worked out much of the biology of Rous sarcoma virus.

Hancock, Joan: Neighbor in Palo Alto who became a lifelong friend.

Haynes, Joel: Scientist at Agracetus who helped develop use of gene gun.

Hellerstein, Michael: Employee of GeoVax who handled regulatory issues as well as developing and overseeing release assays.

Hildebrand, Don: Cofounder and first CEO of GeoVax, Inc.

Huebner, Robert: Scientist at NIH who was active in President Nixon's war against cancer; Huebner provided interim funding for the chickens at Stanford when Kimber Farms was purchased by DeKalb Ag Research.

Hunt, Larry: Professor from the University of Kentucky who did a sabbatical in my lab at the time of the first DNA vaccine experiments.

Insel, Tom: Director of the Yerkes Primate Center who hired me to head the Division of Microbiology and Immunology.

Glossary of Key Contributors

Jameel, Shahid: Established and led the Virology Group at the International Centre for Genetic Engineering and Biotechnology in New Delhi.

Johnston, Peggy: Director of the HIV Vaccine Research Program within the NIH Division of AIDS.

Johnston, Stephen: Pioneer in DNA vaccines and the use of the gene gun.

Keister, Mark: Early employee of GeoVax who handled contracting and regulatory submissions.

LaChaise, Gaston: American sculptor for *Standing Woman*, whom I verbally defended when working at the 1959 American Exhibition in Moscow.

Lamkirt, Olga: Russian émigré who used children's songs and rhymes to teach spoken as well as written Russian. She taught Russian at Swarthmore college.

Lamoureux, Will: Lead scientist at Kimber Farms who facilitated the move of the chickens to Stanford at the time Kimber Farms was acquired by DeKalb Ag Research.

Latham, Dave: Brother who thrived on the Sunday afternoon get-togethers of our eight boys (his five sons and my three sons) to play hockey or baseball (depending on the season) and to eat Sunday dinner together.

Latham, Ginger: The wife of Dave, with whom I cooked on Sunday afternoons for family dinners. Ginger obtained her MD after having a family and by the end of her career had become Director of the Massachusetts Medical Society.

Latham, Nick: My brother who directed Camp Kabeyun and who welcomed the boys not only as campers but as pre-camp handymen.

Latham, Tom: My California brother who came for weekly meals after the senior Bill Robinson had left us. A lawyer, he helped me minimize the expenses of a divorce.

Liu, Margaret: The lead scientist at Merck Inc. for DNA vaccine development.

Lu, Shan: A Howard Hughes fellow who played a seminal role in my lab in the early days of DNA vaccine development. Shan is now a professor at the University of Massachusetts Medical School.

Majno, Guido: Chair of the Department of Pathology at U. Mass medical school who hired me as a research professor and provided interim support in the early days of DNA vaccines when this new technology was not accepted by the greater scientific world.

Mastro, Tim: Key player in developing plans for testing our clade AG HIV vaccine through Projet RETRO-CI in Ivory Coast. At the time of his work with us, he was at the CDC.

McClure, Harold: Veterinarian at Yerkes who provided invaluable expertise and help for trials in nonhuman primates.

Merigan, Tom: Chief of Infectious Diseases at Stanford University, Merigan hired the senior Bill Robinson to join a program bringing molecular approaches to studying and controlling infectious disease. He was critical for securing space for the chickens at Stanford.

Miller, Zell: Politician who, when he was Governor of Georgia, set up the Georgia Research Alliance to attract biotech into Georgia. This program enabled the establishment of the Emory Vaccine Research Center, the institution that I joined when I moved to Georgia. It also established the incubator facility that was the first home of GeoVax.

Moss, Bernie: Director of the Laboratory of Viral Diseases and the NIH Genetic Engineering Section who is an expert on poxviruses, his laboratory provided the MVA vaccines used to boost the DNA vaccines to develop an HIV vaccine.

Nachtrieb, Ellen: Neighbor in Palo Alto who became a long-term friend.

Nixon, Richard: The then vice president of the United States who debated Khruschev at the 1959 Exhibition in Moscow.

Nkengasong, John: Scientist who led Project-RETRO-CI and conducted early trials on anti-HIV drugs in the control of perinatal infections. Nkengasong currently leads PEPFAR.

Penman, Sheldon: Physicist who trained in Darnell's lab and became a leading cellular and molecular biologist, his academic home was MIT.

Robinson, Al: Middle son, born October 7, 1968.

Robinson, Bill: Bill senior, former spouse after whom my eldest son is named.

Robinson, Billy: Oldest son, born August 30, 1967. Billy became Bill when he entered high school.

Robinson, Tom: Youngest son, born November 2, 1969.

Rous, Peyton: Professor at Rockefeller University who first isolated a filterable agent that could cause tumors. The agent became Rous sarcoma virus. Rous won the Nobel Prize for his discovery.

Rubin, Harry: Postdoctoral mentor at the Virus Laboratory, University of California, Berkeley. Rubin worked with Rous sarcoma and its helper viruses.

Salazar, Rick: Employee of Kimber Farms whom I hired to help with the chickens at Stanford and who came to Massachusetts for two months to help set up my first laboratory, at the Worcester Foundation. He was key to the successful move of the chickens and lab.

Santoro, Joe: Senior technician who helped pioneer DNA vaccines.

Schultz, Alan: NIAID officer who oversaw nonhuman primate resources for the Division of AIDS. Schultz arranged for the nonhuman primates used in our first macaque trial.

Sharma, Manju: Secretary, Department of Biotechnology, in the Indian Ministry of Science and Technology who was interested in testing our clade C HIV Vaccine in India.

Shea, Eunice: Live-in-housekeeper who was with us from shortly after our arrival in Massachusetts until the boys were in high school. She became a part of the family.

Smith, Jim: Post-doctoral fellow who was instrumental in making the clade B DNA vaccines for HIV that would go into human trials.

Tannenberg, Walt: Long-standing boyfriend who courted me before marriage and when my marriage broke up, reappeared to spend time not only with me, but also the boys.

Temin, Howard: One of the discoverers of reverse transcriptase.

Tollman, Jan: College roommate who became a long-term friend and travel companion. Tollman is her maiden name.

Vlaming: Woman who provided babysitting for the boys after we returned from sabbatical and needed someone who could drive.

Webster, Rob: Tested early vaccines for avian flu under BSL-4 containment at St. Jude's Hospital in Memphis.

Wolf, Jon: Conducted experiments showing that naked (non-liposome-encapsulated) DNA could be taken up and expressed by muscle cells. His work was done at the University of Wisconsin and licensed by Vical, a San Diego biotech.

Wyatt. Linda: Staff scientist in Bernie Moss's laboratory at the NIAID who made the MVA vaccines that would be used as boosts for our DNA vaccines.

About the Author

Harriet Latham Robinson, born in Boston, attended Girls' Latin School and then Swarthmore College where she majored in Biology. During her Swarthmore years she learned sufficient Russian to obtain a job as a Russian-speaking guide at the 1959 American Exhibition in Moscow. Returning from Russia, she obtained a Masters in Biochemistry and then a Ph.D. in Microbiology at the Massachusetts Institute of Technology, graduating in 1965. Post-doctoral studies at the University of California, Berkeley were followed by marriage and time out to raise three sons to school age.

Re-entering science in 1977, she became a Principal Scientist at the Worcester Foundation for Experimental Biology, served as a Professor of Pathology at the University of Massachusetts Medical School and ultimately became the Asa Griggs Candler Professor and Chief of the Division of Microbiology and Immunology at the Yerkes National Primate Research Center at Emory University. Dr. Robinson is internationally recognized for her early studies on insertional mutagenesis and oncogene transduction in retroviral-induced cancers, her pioneering studies on the use of recombinant DNA for vaccination, and her recent work towards an HIV/AIDS vaccine. In 2001 she co-founded GeoVax Inc, a company formed to help take her candidate AIDS vaccine into human clinical trials.

Printed in Great Britain
by Amazon